NutriSystem Nourish

NutriSystem Nourish

The Revolutionary New Weight-Loss Program

NutriSystem
and Dr. James Rouse

WILEY

John Wiley & Sons, Inc.

Published by John Wiley & Sons, Inc., Hoboken, New Jersey
Published simultaneously in Canada

Design and production by Navta Associates, Inc.

For general information about our other products and services, please contact our Customer Care Department within the United States at (800) 762-2974, outside the United States at (317) 572-3993 or fax (317) 572-4002.

Wiley also publishes its books in a variety of electronic formats. Some content that appears in print may not be available in electronic books. For more information about Wiley products, visit our web site at www.wiley.com.

Library of Congress Cataloging-in-Publication Data

NutriSystem nourish : the revolutionary new weight-loss program :
NutriSystem and Dr. James Rouse.
    p. cm.
  Includes index.
  ISBN 0-471-65365-9 (cloth : alk. paper)
1. Weight loss. I. Rouse, James, 1963–
  RM222.2.N88 2004
  613.2'5—dc22

                                              2004000432

Printed in the United States of America

10 9 8 7 6 5 4 3 2 1

Contents

v

Acknowledgments

This book is the co-creative effort of many gifted people.

First, I would like to thank my wife, Debra, for being my best friend, editor extraordinaire, and the type of person we all dream of in a life partner. Thanks, also, to my two beautiful girls, Dakota and Elli, for your hugs, laughter, and unconditional acceptance of your daddy and his time taken on the computer. And thanks to my parents, for giving me a foundation of love and the inner compass of belief to go after my heart's longings. I'd also like to thank the family at NutriSystem—it truly has been a blessing to be enveloped by such a loving and supportive group of amazing people who always come from the heart.

Special thanks to editor Beth VanderVennet for her expertise, and also to nutritionist Robin Rifkin, M.S., for creating all of the wonderful NutriSystem Nourish recipes, to Dr. Jay Satz for his profound weight-loss expertise, to Mary Gregg, Registered Dietitian, for her nutritional contributions, and to Ele Fisher for her help with the jacket design.

Thanks to George Jankovic, Delphine Carroll, and Sheri Keiles for putting their arms around this project and ensuring a quality product; and to Mike Hagan for his sheer and absolute faith in me.

Thanks also to Jeffrey Brous, Cathy Cassidy, Shannon Crossin, Patrick Miller, Charles Plyter, Theresa Suevo and the rest of the team at NutriSystem.

I would also like to thank Tom Miller and the entire staff at Wiley for their knowledge, encouragement, and help in bringing this book to life. They have played an integral role in bringing hope and nourishment to countless lives for years to come.

And last, I wish to thank all of my patients and clients who have taught me about healing. You have blessed me with the experience of witnessing how through loving and accepting yourselves, you can transform not only your own lives, but also the lives of those around you. It has been an honor—thank you!

—Dr. James Rouse

NutriSystem Nourish

Introduction

Welcome to the revolutionary weight-loss program designed to jumpstart your metabolism and give you breakthrough weight-loss results.

Welcome to a healthy new weight-loss program that emphasizes low-glycemic carbs, an optimal amount of protein and healthy fats, and a mind–body approach to weight loss that will help you lose weight as you never have been able to before.

Welcome to a simple-to-follow weight-loss program that's easy to incorporate into your busy lifestyle and that will be your catalyst to living the life you've always dreamed about.

Welcome to NutriSystem Nourish!

Do you want to lose weight once and for all? Would you like to find a way to drop unwanted pounds that actually fits into your lifestyle? How about feeling great—really great—about yourself once again, and putting the past behind you and envisioning a whole new future? All of these things are possible through this new, innovative program, and I'm here to tell you all about it.

I am a naturopathic physician and director of coordinated care and complementary medicine at the Phoenix Center for Health Excellence. For years, at my clinical practice in Denver, Colorado, I've worked with patients who want to lose weight. I've had people come to me who have needed to lose 20, 40, or even as many as 140 pounds. Aside from most of them losing at least 6 to 13 pounds in just the first 2 weeks, they've continued safely losing 1 to 2½ pounds each week thereafter and they've been able to keep the weight off for the long term—something most diets these days can't deliver. What's the secret?

From working with such a wide variety of people over the years, interestingly enough, it always comes down to one simple thing that's key to losing weight: in order to do it, you must manage your life and yourself. In other words, weight loss isn't just about pounds, it's about people—including everything that makes us tick.

Certainly, if you want to lose weight, what's going into your mouth matters; but what's going on in your brain and in the lifestyle you choose matters just as much, particularly if you're aiming for long-term weight management. In order to lose weight, you need to manage both the physical and mental aspects of the weight-loss process. Key concepts must be addressed, understood, and taken to heart in order to succeed. That's why I wrote this book.

This approach works—I know it, my patients know it, and the people at NutriSystem know it. For more than 30 years, NutriSystem has been helping people lose weight. Together we created this new and breakthrough weight-loss program that can work for you, even if you lead a busy life. By combining the latest nutrition and scientific research that's behind the new NutriSystem Nourish product line with movement and the hormonal body chemistry and behavioral expertise that I've been perfecting with my patients for years, the revolutionary new NutriSystem Nourish program has come to life, and it's already completely changing the way thousands of people approach the task of losing weight. It's The Good Carb Answer™, and the most well-rounded weight-loss program on the market today, as it embraces the notion that to achieve significant weight-loss results, you need to fuel all aspects of the self. Through its specially formulated meal plans, explicit exercise program, and motivational mindset tools, it delivers complete nourishment for the total you. With this plan, everything comes together and you lose weight.

This approach has worked for my patients and for countless others pleased with their success on the NutriSystem program. In a recent survey of current NutriSystem customers, 95 percent of them said they would recommend the NutriSystem program to a friend. And this book shows you practical ways to implement the same comprehensive weight-loss plan into your own busy lifestyle, on your own terms, to make it work for *you*. It's my hope, my dream, to share this insight with you so that you can succeed, too.

You can plan on losing up to 17 pounds in just 4 weeks on this program by simply following its low-glycemic meal plans, exercise initiatives, and new lifestyle techniques. It's all there, waiting for you to begin!

I don't know your unique story, but chances are that at some point you have been on a one-dimensional diet plan built on deprivation, where scarcity is the ruling mantra. These plans are usually only temporary, lasting just long enough to get your weight down before you inevitably return to your old life patterns. These diets can leave you feeling fatigued and irritable or fighting ravenous cravings, depression, or other less-than-compelling experiences. These symptoms are very common among dieters because most programs do not take into account the human need for fulfillment—for that innate need to thrive and achieve true success. This program does. That's what separates the new NutriSystem Nourish program from other "diets." This innovative program sees weight loss differently and considers the bigger picture of what eating well and losing weight can look like: less weight, boundless energy, restful sleep, increased endurance, greater optimism, and greater joy. It's a total mentality shift that views pounds lost as life gained.

On the NutriSystem Nourish program, you will definitely lose weight and keep losing until you reach your goal. But more importantly, on this program you'll also gain an entirely new way of thinking and living, which will be key to keeping the weight off. I want to share with you, up front, exactly what you can expect to gain from this program and learn from this book.

Chapter 1, "Food Is Fuel for Life: Nourish to Flourish," launches the book and addresses nutrition as it applies to your body's ability to lose weight. I start with this topic because food is so vital in all of our lives, yet so many of us now see it as public (and private) enemy #1. But now it's time to view food as fuel for your body to burn. Learn all about good carbs and bad carbs and how they affect your ability to lose weight. What's the glycemic index, and what does it have to do with whether your pants fit you this season? You'll find out the answers to these questions in Chapter 1, as well as learn how protein can minimize the effects of a decadent dessert, which kinds of cookies are kindest to your hips, and what green tea can do for your waistline. This program is The Good Carb Answer, and in this chapter, I'll tell you why.

Chapter 2, "Tuning Your Metabolic Machinery: Fixing a Slow

Metabolism," takes things one step further and explains how nutrition affects your metabolism. Did you ever think you could actually program your own metabolism and not just be stuck with the one you were born with? You can, and in Chapter 2 you'll find out exactly how to choose the one you want. Is snacking good for your weight-loss efforts? Which is worse for your body: peanut M&Ms or jelly beans? Find out in this chapter, along with more specifics on how your blood sugar levels affect your metabolism, and what your hormones have to do with weight loss and health. We'll also discuss how skipping meals and depriving yourself of regular nutrition can sabotage your metabolism. Plus you'll get five quick and fun Metabolic Minute exercises you can do to rev up your body throughout the day. It's all about tuning up your metabolic machine, and by the end of this chapter, you'll have all the tools you need to burn, baby, burn!

Chapter 3, "Mind Over Matter: Losing Weight Without Losing Your Mind," takes your weight-loss efforts up a notch, into your head. This is where we integrate the crucial mind component into your weight-loss plan, and it's what makes this plan unique and different from all those other diets out there. In this chapter, you'll see why sometimes it really is all in your head, and you'll begin to understand your mind's role in the weight-loss process. Are you suffering from "overdoingitis" and have you used your "mental floss" lately? After reading this chapter, you'll know how to answer those questions and incorporate "But" Reduction into your weight-loss regime. When it comes to weight loss, our thoughts and beliefs can make us our own worst enemies. But by the end of Chapter 3, you'll see that whereas willpower is a thing of the past, your willingness is where it's all at now. Where there's a will, there's a weigh.

Chapter 4, "Relax Your Mind, Shrink Your Behind: The Stress/Fat Connection," is where I address stress and its impact on your weight-loss efforts. It's true—if you relax your mind, it *will* help shrink your behind— but do you know how? Learn what the hormone cortisol is and whether it's your weight-loss friend or foe. And exactly what does stress have to do with how your body burns fat? In this chapter, you'll find out. Plus, I provide you with easy, concrete ways to relax and focus on the day at hand so that you can reduce stress. Can you spare 1 minute or maybe 5 during your day to reduce stress? Then I've got nourishing mind exercises for you. Can you find maybe 20 or 30 minutes to decompress? One breath at a time, you'll learn to recreate your entire daily experience. Things like deep breathing and meditation aren't just for the ultra–New Age or extremely serene anymore.

Is stress really fattening? By the end of this chapter, you'll have your answer as well as concrete tools for managing it.

In Chapter 5, the "NutriSystem Nourish Meal Plans" come to life. By this point, you've read about food, your metabolism, and the role your mind and stress play in weight loss, and it's time to dive into the heart of the NutriSystem Nourish program—the meal plans. In this section, you'll get 28 days of simple and practical NutriSystem Nourish meal plans. These are the foundation of the NutriSystem Nourish program and what you may typically look for when you begin any weight-loss initiative—what's the plan, what am I going to get to eat, and how often? You'll notice that you get to eat five times a day and that you'll be enjoying a variety of foods, including fruits and vegetables, as well as foods containing good carbohydrates and optimal levels of proteins. You'll also notice right away that it's a simple and easy-to-follow program and that it's not one of those extreme plans where you knock out whole food groups or go super high or low anything. This plan is all about variety and balance. You eat foods you prepare yourself in the Do-It-Yourself Meal Plan or those handy foods already prepared for you by NutriSystem in the Prepared Foods Meal Plan, and follow a simple schedule that kicks in your metabolism so that you can lose weight—up to 13 pounds in the first 2 weeks and up to 2½ pounds each week after that. Just follow the program and you'll start losing weight.

Chapter 6, "Move It to Lose It: You Choose—Xercise or Xtra Size?" begins Part III, which is our exercise section, and it's where we tackle fitness and your attitude toward fitness. The human body was designed to move, and moving is especially important if you want to burn fat, but exercise doesn't have to be a chore. I give you fun, easy ways to incorporate movement into your life even if you can only find 10 or 15 minutes in your day to exercise. I also answer questions: When's the best time of day to exercise? Which is better for encouraging weight loss: walking or jogging? Should you consider lifting weights if you are older than 50? Plus, you'll see how exercise affects things like your hormones and your energy level. Exercise doesn't have to be something you dread. It can be something you look forward to because it's one of your greatest allies in the battle of the bulge. By the end of this chapter, you'll *want* to exercise!

Chapter 7, "The NutriSystem Nourish Exercise Plan: Your Choose-to-Move Program," naturally fits right here, and in this chapter you'll find a 4-week exercise plan that you can use whether you're a beginner, intermediate, or advanced exerciser. I personally put these routines together and believe they are an excellent fitness program for anyone looking to increase his or her metabolism and lose weight. I outline exactly what your daily exercise program should be and walk you through each movement and exercise. There are also helpful photos of people doing the actual exercises with me, and it's simple to follow along. This chapter will be your fitness guide as you introduce or reintroduce movement into your life.

Chapter 8, "Steps to Success: Resolve to Evolve," wraps everything up. You'll find the five steps to NutriSystem Nourish, the key elements that form the foundation of the program and your success. I share with you all the wonderful reasons why you will succeed on this program and tell you a little bit about all the wonderful kinds of support you can get from the NutriSystem Nourish program. This is where everything gels and where you learn to put the NutriSystem Nourish program—the meal plans, exercise routines, and lifestyle practices—into motion. You'll feel empowered to go forward and make everything you desire happen.

Chapter 9, "NutriSystem Nourish Recipes," is an amazing culinary resource. Just when you thought we couldn't fit anything more into this book, you'll find 75 easy-to-prepare recipes, all designed to help you lose weight. From Southwestern Meatloaf and Black Bean Stew to Flan and Creamy Baked Cheesecake with Blueberry Topping, we've gathered some of our best-tasting dishes and created them with nutritious ingredients so that you get a delicious blend of hearty and healthy low-glycemic foods to enjoy throughout your entire program. With the NutriSystem Nourish recipes you'll feel like you have your own healthy chef alongside you in the kitchen. You'll never be hungry again!

It's truly a joy to share this book and all of its wonderful ideas and information with you. By the time you're through reading it, you'll have practical ideas and methods for getting your body and mindset primed for weight loss. Most importantly, you'll have all the tools you need to start losing weight right now.

Life is busy, and I know your time is at a premium. But how much you weigh and how you feel about yourself affects your entire life and the way you operate in the world; it's fundamental to your happiness and how well you experience everything in your life. It's well worth your valuable time and energy to learn how to manage your weight successfully by following the best program you can find. Now you've found it, so you can begin!

This NutriSystem Nourish program is the weight-loss breakthrough you've been searching for—your means to looking great, feeling great, and discovering ultimate freedom in your life. When it comes to losing weight, it's your choice—you can either do something new that will work for you or you can continue down the same old path that brought you here in the first place. It's up to you.

Right now, you hold two things in your hands: your future and this book. Why not let them both work for you?

Join me. It's time to Nourish!

PART ONE

Nourishing Weight Loss

1

Food Is Fuel for Life
Nourish to Flourish

We think about food *way too much*.

We overthink our daily food choices on a routine basis, making things increasingly difficult on ourselves. It's why more than half of us are overweight, and almost all of us struggle to maintain a healthy weight. As a society, our favorite three words seem to be *What's for dinner?* while we're constantly mustering up all the willpower we can to avoid overeating and bingeing.

Your head tells you one thing—that carrot sticks would be a much better choice than that half-gallon of cherry chocolate chip ice cream—but your habits take you down a different path and you're stuck once again. It seems impossible to find direction, let alone the strength to go on.

I know. I've seen this struggle firsthand with my patients, over and over again. This constant battle with what we eat has turned food into nothing shy of a four-letter word. But no longer!

Starting today, we're looking at food as fuel and as a tool to help you lose weight. We're going to learn about it and use it to get the best mileage we can out of life.

The Need for Nutrition

Anytime you consider starting a weight-loss program, the big question is, What do I get to eat? Pasta? Desserts? Snacks? Wine? You're probably wondering the same thing about this program, and while it's tempting to jump ahead and fill you in on the exciting, new NutriSystem Nourish meal plan we've put together, let me tell you that you get to eat all those great-tasting things—plus a whole lot more.

Food is important to us, especially when we're trying to lose weight, and when viewed as fuel, it takes on even more significance in our lives. Questions like what kind of this should I eat and how much of that should I have trouble us every day, and it seems almost weekly there's some new study unveiling the latest pros and cons about the foods we eat. We're constantly surrounded by food issues and difficult choices, and sometimes just knowing what to feed ourselves seems nearly impossible.

That's where the NutriSystem Nourish program comes in. It outlines exactly what and how much you should be eating, so there's no more guesswork or risk of making bad choices. We designed it to help eliminate doubt and to ensure that while you're losing weight, you're also meeting all of your nutritional needs. It's intended to create a level of body chemistry excellence that encourages weight loss—up to 6 to 13 pounds in just the first 2 weeks—by fostering hormonal blood sugar balance, which in turn maximizes your metabolism, increases your energy, lowers your stress, and supports your peace of mind. This plan works!

Through this program, you have a choice between cooking your own dishes (you'll learn to prepare healthy meals, and we have 75 delicious recipes in this book) and eating great-tasting NutriSystem prepared foods—or even enjoying whatever combination of the two works for you. You'll find that this program fits beautifully into a busy lifestyle and jump-starts your body so that it starts burning fat more efficiently, which means more weight loss for you.

Your body chemistry is designed to thrive. That's why successful weight loss, sustained energy, and optimal well-being can all be attained by getting the right amounts of vitamins, minerals, and nutrients. By following the NutriSystem Nourish program that's centered around good, solid nutrition, weight loss is the natural progression.

You will learn to change the types of foods you're eating to include more whole foods and fewer processed foods. You will monitor your sugars and unhealthy fats, and you'll learn to make better carbohydrate choices.

A Day in the Life of NutriSystem Nourish

Luann uses a combination of the Prepared Foods Meal Plan and the Do-It-Yourself Meal Plan for her weight-loss program.

Luann is a working woman who lives with her 8-year-old daughter and wants to lose 40 pounds. It's Tuesday, and her alarm goes off at

6 A.M. Slowly she heads toward her favorite comfy chair for 10 minutes of deep breathing while focusing positively on the day ahead of her. From there, she hops on the treadmill in her laundry room for a 20-minute walk before hitting the shower. By 7:15, she's eating breakfast with her daughter (a bowl of NutriSystem Low-Fat Granola with banana slices and a glass of fat-free milk), and they're out the door by 8 A.M.

Luann's morning flies by and by 11:30 she's ready for her lunch including NutriSystem Hearty Minestrone Soup and the salad she fixed last night. She tops her meal off with some key lime yogurt and heads out the door with a coworker for a 10-minute walk around the office complex to complete her lunch hour. At 3 P.M., she snacks on an apple and low-fat string cheese at her desk, and while heading out her office door, she practices her Doorway Exercise as she's done all day when passing through thresholds—she repeats her affirmation, "I want to be strong, healthy, and vibrant, and I have the power to make this happen in my life."

By 6 P.M., Luann is home with her daughter, preparing home-cooked Turkey Tostadas (from the NutriSystem Nourish recipes) and helping her daughter with homework in the kitchen. By 8:30, after paying some bills, she sits down to enjoy a NutriSystem Mochaccino Dessert Bar while thinking about what she's going to wear to work the next day.

It's been another great day on the NutriSystem Nourish program for Luann.

The Carb/Sugar Connection

The new NutriSystem Nourish program views food as fuel. It's there to provide power for your life. And one major source of this fuel is carbohydrates.

I know that there are many diets out there talking about low-carb or no-carb approaches, and that for many people carb has actually become a fearsome foe. But I'm not willing to feed this fear of carbohydrates. Instead, I'm going to let you in on why this plan is The Good Carb Answer. I'm going to tell you about some good carb choices and encourage you to eat the right kinds of carbohydrates that will support your metabolism, your mood, and your overall health and well-being. By avoiding the bad carbohydrates, you will lose weight.

The #1 thing you need to know about all carbohydrates is that they have a direct connection to insulin in your body, and that insulin affects the way you gain weight. Your pancreas produces the hormone insulin in response to an increase of sugar in the bloodstream. When your pancreas notices that the level of sugar in your body has suddenly risen, such as after you've eaten some ice cream or a cookie, it kicks in and sends out insulin to help your body utilize the sugar for energy. When this insulin is sent out, it converts the sugar to glycogen, which your body needs and stores in your liver for later use. However, only so much of that glycogen can be stored up, and once those stores become full, the rest of the sugar that's being converted has nowhere to go, yet the insulin continues converting it—at this point, into *fat*.

Once those stores are full, your body and all fat-burning systems shut down and all you do is *store fat*—the very fat that keeps you from fitting into those favorite jeans. And in addition to adding inches to your waistline, this storage of fat affects your body in other detrimental ways, like decreasing the release of your muscle-building hormones, weakening your immune system, and raising cholesterol and triglycerides—all a direct result of consuming too much sugar.

That's why balancing your blood sugar levels—something you can do through the NutriSystem Nourish program—is so key. This includes carbohydrates, too, because as they're metabolized, carbohydrates are converted by your body into sugar, which enters your bloodstream to be used as energy. It's imperative to choose good ones—those carbs that are metabolized slowly into sugar—because they enter the bloodstream more slowly, which keeps your blood sugar levels normal, so you don't send out too much insulin and start storing fat.

Good carbs = normal sugar and insulin levels
= less fat stored and less hunger

Now you can see why we're on the hunt for the kind of carbohydrates that trigger the least amount of insulin to be released, so fat doesn't get stored. These are good carbs and there's a simple way to find out what foods they're in.

All Carbs Are Not Created Equal

Somewhere along the line, researchers began testing foods and carbohydrates to see how various types were quickly broken down into sugar, then absorbed into the bloodstream. They knew that the more slowly a carb breaks down as sugar the better, because then it doesn't spike your insulin

Good Carb, Bad Carb

This chart shows the effect that eating low-glycemic carbohydrates has on your blood sugar levels versus when you consume high-glycemic carbohydrates. Remember, the more insulin that your body releases, the more fat it stores.

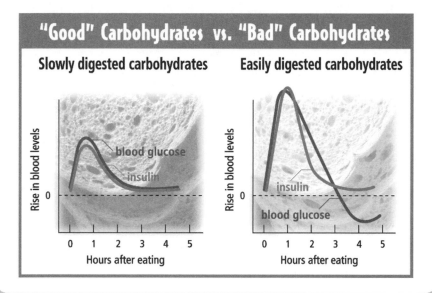

level as much and encourage the storage of fat. From their research they established a ranking of carbohydrates in foods based on their effect on blood sugar, and they called it the glycemic index (see Appendix).

Those carbohydrates that broke down slowly were given a lower number on the glycemic index and were identified as better for the body. Those carbohydrates that broke down more quickly and caused insulin levels to spike and fat to be stored were given a higher number on the index and identified as worse for the body.

Although two meals may contain the same number of carbohydrates (in grams), they might actually produce quite different effects on blood sugar and sugar levels in the body, depending on whether good or bad carbs were eaten. This is extremely important for all of us to know—especially those who are overweight or have high triglycerides, diabetes, or syndrome X (insulin resistance). With the exception of elite endurance athletes, carbohydrates that have a high-glycemic-index value are a problem for anyone trying to burn fat, optimize energy levels, and lower cholesterol. The World Health Organization recommends that people in industrialized countries base their diets on low-glycemic-index foods in order to prevent the most common diseases of affluence, such as coronary heart disease, diabetes, and obesity.

The higher the glycemic index of the food, the quicker the lift—and the faster the fall. And when your blood sugar levels drop, you feel hungry. That is why it is important to maintain normal blood sugar levels. For long-burning, sustained energy, you need to choose foods with lower-glycemic-index values, as we did when creating the new NutriSystem Nourish program. By doing so, you will find it easier to lose weight, since carbohydrates will be used up for energy in fueling your body and your metabolism, rather than being stored as fat.

Cookie Catastrophe

Do you crave or eat cookies a little too often? If you're a cookie person, all the wheels do not need to come off when you indulge in your favorite treat. Instead, do these things to keep from creating a total dietary disaster:

- Choose to use whole grains when making cookies.
- Use oats instead of flour in your cookies.
- Add oat bran to your mix.
- Add nuts to your mix.
- Have a protein portion before you eat your cookie.

Examples of good low-glycemic food choices are fresh fruit, green vegetables, multigrain breads, sweet potatoes, broccoli, all-bran cereals, regular oatmeal, and even pasta cooked al dente. Examples of high-glycemic foods to avoid include white bread, mashed potatoes, white rice, and corn flakes. (See the Appendix for a complete listing of glycemic index values.)

Nourish No-Cheat Sheet

Here are quick ways to help balance your blood sugar levels even if you're eating sweets:

- Add protein powder to your whole-grain pancakes, cookies, cupcakes, and smoothies.
- Add fiber to your baking mixes or sprinkle wheat germ or ground flax on top of your meals to cushion the sugar response before you indulge.
- Have a serving of protein along with or before your dessert to help keep blood sugar and insulin more balanced.

The good news is that the entire new NutriSystem Nourish program is based on lower-glycemic-index foods. That's why the plan is referred to as The Good Carb Answer. So whether you're cooking for yourself or enjoying prepared NutriSystem meals, you'll get the right amount of good carbs to fuel your body when you follow the program.

Why Low-Glycemic Carbs Are Better Than No Carbs

At this point, you might be asking if you should just avoid carbs altogether. Many of my patients ask me this. It is the concept behind most of the no-carb/high-protein diets out there nowadays, but this type of thinking is flawed. A low-glycemic meal plan is far better for weight loss than simply avoiding all carbs for the following reasons:

- Carbohydrates are a direct source of energy and your body needs them to fuel its metabolism.
- A very low-carb diet is difficult to stay on for any length of time because you like carbs and your body craves them.
- The high-fat content in most low-carb diets can cause yo-yo dieting, and the long-term effects of this lifestyle can seriously affect your health.
- Low-carb diets don't provide enough direct energy, so your body is instead forced to burn protein—muscle mass—for fuel, which hampers weight loss and actually slows down your metabolism.

Additionally, research shows that low-glycemic-index carbohydrates contain key compounds critical in fighting various diseases including cancer. Good carbohydrates like the ones incorporated into the NutriSystem Nourish program not only benefit your metabolism and fat burning processes but also carry significant amounts of phytonutrients and antioxidants, which are powerful disease-fighting compounds. Your body needs these nutrients, and if stripped of its source of them, it will struggle to fight disease.

How a Low-Glycemic-Index Meal Plan Keeps You from Feeling Hungry

I am sure one of the major questions still on your mind is if the NutriSystem Nourish program can control your hunger. The answer is an overwhelming yes. My patients have told me time and time again that while they were losing weight on a low-glycemic plan they were amazed at how they didn't feel hungry. The reason is that low-glycemic carbohydrate foods stay in your intestines longer, which tells your brain that you are full for a longer period of time. Low-glycemic carbohydrate meals help to control your blood sugar level, which also reduces your feeling of hunger throughout the day. Through its low-glycemic carbohydrates and proper balance of proteins and fats, the NutriSystem Nourish meal plan is your best weapon against hunger.

Fiber's Role in Weight Loss

Fiber also is key to nutrition and weight loss for the same reason those good carbs are: it helps keep your insulin levels low. In fact, most fiber-rich foods have a low-glycemic-index value, so they play a vital role in helping you slow down the speed in which sugar enters the bloodstream.

By eating a balance of high-fiber, low-glycemic carbohydrates, you slow your sugar absorption and lower your insulin, thus encouraging your metabolic best to help you lose weight. Adding fiber and protein to your meal lowers its total glycemic level. Fiber supplies the bulk in your diet and can aid in lowering cholesterol levels and preventing constipation, hemorrhoids, and heart disease. Fiber-rich foods are more satisfying to your body's natural system for registering a feeling of fullness. When you eat foods rich in fiber, satiety—or that feeling of being satisfied after a meal—is achieved earlier and lasts longer than when you eat refined foods, which tend to have higher glycemic values. Fiber-rich foods help to slow the breakdown of blood sugars, making you feel less hungry.

Getting Enough Fiber in Your Diet

When it comes to fiber, your goal should be to consume at least 25 to 30 grams of it each day from a variety of different food sources—which may be a little trickier than it sounds. Today, most of our grains are stripped of their fiber. They are processed and refined in a process that removes the fibrous bran and beneficial oils. Through the NutriSystem Nourish meal plan, you'll be following a program that lets you eat whole foods like fresh fruits, vegetables, and whole grains, which ensures that you are getting enough fiber in your diet. Consumed in their natural state, these delicious foods can help provide your daily dose of nutritious, health-affirming fiber and offer protection against a variety of chronic diseases. Whole foods found in the NutriSystem Nourish plan are good sources of soluble fiber, which serves your body well by creating a sticky gel that acts like a protective coating to prevent harmful substances from doing damage. A recent major university study found that men who ate 7 grams of soluble fiber daily were 40 percent less likely to die from heart disease than those getting only 4 grams. Great soluble fiber sources include prunes, avocados, black beans, kidney beans, artichokes, sweet potatoes, figs, and apples.

Insoluble fiber is another form of fiber that comes from the supportive structural material of plants. It stimulates normal movement in the intestinal tract and can dilute the concentration of toxins that may be residing in the colon. This type of fiber can also prevent the formation of diverticulosis, a disease involving the intestinal wall. Great insoluble fiber sources include avocados, blackberries, guava, wheat bran, prunes, lentils, broccoli, brussels sprouts, mung beans, and carrots.

One other thing that's important to mention when we're talking about fiber is water. Everyone knows that water is a must for ultimate weight loss. It moistens and lubricates our tissues and joints, helps eliminate wastes and toxins from our tissues, and is crucial in our body's ability to transport vital nutrients, proteins, sugars, electrolytes, minerals, and vitamins for proper assimilation. A reasonable goal is to drink eight 8-ounce glasses daily. Another way to calculate your individual needs is to divide your body weight in half and drink that amount in ounces. When you increase the amount of fiber in your diet, you need to increase your intake of water, too. Fiber acts much like a sponge in your system, soaking up fluids in your body, which causes an increased need to adequately hydrate all the cells so that they can do their best work.

When you increase your fiber intake, you also want to prevent any blockage from occurring. You want to make sure the fiber remains well lubricated and slippery so that it can pass entirely through your system, grabbing debris along the way and not getting stuck somewhere in your intestines. Water binds with the fiber in your meals, increasing its thickness and making it more bulky. This delays the transit time through your intestinal tract, slowing digestion and absorption of carbohydrates.

The Word on Protein

You can't talk about nutrition or weight loss these days without talking about protein. It's a hot topic and an essential element for creating balance and serving as the building block for muscle tissue. Protein is vital for immunity, proper hormone balance, and enzyme synthesis. What does it have to do with weight loss?

Like good carbs and fiber, protein also helps to balance blood sugar levels, but it does so in a different way. Protein is an activator for the release of glucagon. What is glucagon? It's another hormone secreted by the pancreas that helps regulate blood sugar and promotes the mobilization of previously stored fat. Glucagon plays an opposite role to that of insulin, and it helps the body mobilize fat for burning, to be used as a fuel source. Optimal protein equals more glucagon, which means increased fat burning.

That's why many recent diets have encouraged high protein consumption in an effort to mobilize the fat-burning process even more. But many high-protein diets have gone too far. These diets are hard to stick with due to many factors, including cravings and a low hormonal balance, which can contribute to mood and emotional swings that can undermine the positive effects of a balanced weight-loss plan. The safety of these diets is also questionable. Long-term studies on the dangers of high-protein diets have not yet been done, although we do know that excessive protein in the diet has already been linked to many health challenges including osteoporosis and kidney problems.

On the other end of the spectrum, low-protein diets challenge your ability to lose weight, too, due to excessive insulin levels and blood sugar imbalances. Both of these extremes can foster weight gain and cravings.

How Much Protein Is Enough?

To encourage a healthy lifestyle and support fat burning—and your ability to keep the weight off in the long run—you need a moderate amount of protein, which is exactly what you get with the NutriSystem Nourish program. It's based on what I recommend to my patients: a protein-adequate eating plan for health. I see great results in clients who consume roughly 25 percent of their daily calories from protein.

All proteins are not created equal in terms of weight loss and health. High-quality proteins can be found in many foods from both animal and vegetable sources. Leaner proteins such as fish, skinless poultry, and lean game meats, as well as soy foods like tofu and tempeh, are less dramatic on the body than heavy steaks and fatty pork, plus they have fewer fat calories.

Chewing the Fat

So far, we've talked about carbohydrates, fiber, and protein and how each of them helps to balance your blood sugar levels and improve your body's ability to lose weight. You've also learned about insulin, the glycemic index, and glucagons. What's left is fat.

In the past few decades, fat has pretty much become its own four-letter word. The tide is changing, though, when it comes to whether it's okay to consume it. It seems that the so-called experts were actually mistaken when they encouraged us to avoid fats. Evidence now shows that we in fact need certain fats to maintain optimal health—and like everything else, when it comes to fats, balance is key.

Fats are required for nearly every process in your body. They operate as an energy source for the body and perform many crucial tasks. They serve as overall insulation and aid in cell membrane integrity, cardiovascular functions, and hormone production. As with carbohydrates, it's the *quality* of fat that you eat that's important and has everything to do with whether it's good or bad for your body. Four of the most prevalent types of fat are omega-6, omega-3, saturated fats, and trans fats.

The good fats are the omega-3 and some omega-6 fatty acids, and they're important to consume, as they're essential for cellular structure and hormone production. But they have to be consumed in moderate amounts to produce their beneficial effects. Researchers at Baker Medical Research Institute in Melbourne, Australia, studied the ability of omega-3 oils from fish to aid in the prevention of hardening of the arteries, a condition that can lead to hypertension, heart attack, and stroke. In the study, published in the *American Journal of Clinical Nutrition,* the group of patients taking a fish oil supplement showed a significant increase in artery softness—a desired effect. The group not receiving the fish oils showed no change. The information concerning the protective effects of fish oils is so powerful that the American Heart Association recommends that you eat at least 6 ounces of fish per week. It appears that these omega-3 fatty acids may offer as much protection against heart disease as the cholesterol-lowering drugs on the market today. We have several menus that include fish and several recipes for fish dishes in the NutriSystem Nourish recipe section. If you don't like fish, you can get omega-3 fats in other seafood or in fish oil capsules.

Research is also discovering that a lack of consumption of omega-3 and other key fats can affect us in a variety of ways. Fat deficiencies can cause a decrease in energy and metabolism, emotional and mental challenges like depression and memory loss, brittle nails and hair, and premature aging of the skin.

Two not-so-great fats are saturated fats and trans fatty acids. Saturated fats are found in many meat and dairy products and should be limited in the diet because they have been linked to diseases such as obesity, cardiovascular disease, and cancer. Additionally, extensive research has shown that trans fatty acids, which are found in meat and dairy and in processed food in the form of partially hydrogenated oils, are twice as likely to cause heart disease and stroke than are saturated fats. Trans fats have been shown to raise low-density lipoproteins (which causes the clogging of blood vessels), and to reduce high-density lipoproteins (which clear blood vessels)—of course, neither effect is good for cardiovascular health. The United States government is so concerned about the consumption of these trans fats that legislation will soon require all nutritional labels to include the quantity per serving of these types of fats contained in the food. Trans fats are especially problematic when consumed in excess, which can happen when you overindulge in highly processed carbohydrate snacks and baked goods.

Munchie Modifications

Sometimes our cravings get the best of us, but there are still good choices to be made. Try these snack-saving suggestions when the munchies attack. Their glycemic values are lower and they'll do a little less damage to your blood sugar level:

- A handful of peanuts instead of pretzels
- A few peanut M&Ms instead of jelly beans
- Mini Snickers instead of Life Savers
- Low-fat chocolate milk instead of ice cream
- Pumpernickel bread instead of a baguette
- Raspberries with chocolate instead of plain chocolate

When it comes to fats, think in with the good, out with the bad, and rest assured, the fats included in the NutriSystem Nourish program have been formulated to help you maintain normal body functioning and to help you lose weight.

Supplements

Although I tend to shy away from arming my clients with an entire arsenal of capsules, tablets, powders, and oils, I definitely am not reserved when it comes to recommending supplements that may improve your state of health and increase your vitality. Many supplements can be useful during and after weight loss.

Multivitamins

A general multivitamin/mineral is indispensable, since most of us fail to acquire all the nutrients we need through foods. I eat an extremely clean, organic, healthful, and low-glycemic-plentiful diet, yet I still make sure to take a high-potency multiple vitamin every day. A multivitamin supplement is inexpensive nutrition insurance. While it will not provide the phytonutrients or fiber of whole foods like fruits and vegetables, a good vitamin supplement does provide 100 percent of the recommended daily allowance (RDA) for the established vitamins and some minerals. While on any weight-loss program, it is a prudent thing to do and I highly recommend it.

However, be wary of and avoid supplements that include megadoses of particular vitamins or minerals, since some of the fat-soluble vitamins are stored in the body (like vitamins A, D, and K) and large amounts of them built up in your body can cause harmful effects over time.

Always check the expiration date when buying supplements. Also look for a USP marking on the label, which indicates that the United States Pharmacopeia has declared that the vitamin actually contains the ingredients in the amounts stated on the label and that the tablets will dissolve effectively. Finally, always be sure to take your vitamin supplement with a meal for best absorption.

Calcium

Besides carbon, hydrogen, oxygen, and nitrogen, calcium is the most abundant mineral in your body. That makes it the most important mineral for your health, and because it is continuously being metabolized and eventually excreted from your body, it must be continually replaced, from the foods you consume.

Beyond calcium's major role of maintaining bone structure and preventing bone loss, it has now been shown to be a major factor in weight loss. Calcium suppresses hormones that promote fat storage and weight gain and actually stimulates the breakdown of fat. To achieve maximum weight loss, your calcium consumption should be at least 1,200 milligrams per day.

And it's important to note that studies have shown that calcium derived from milk produced greater weight loss than that derived from calcium supplements such as calcium carbonate, so while taking a calcium supplement is an option, you should try to consume most of your calcium from calcium-rich whole foods. The NutriSystem Nourish plan includes many of these foods.

Omega-3

As we previously discussed, omega-3 fish oils are important in preventing heart disease. Most of the omega fish oils can be found in dark fish like salmon, tuna, and mackerel, but if you are not eating two servings of fish per week, you should be taking a fish oil supplement.

Green Tea

Green tea has become a very popular drink in North America because there is good evidence that it has antioxidant properties that help reduce the risk of cancer and heart disease. Several recent studies have indicated that green tea can help promote weight loss by burning extra calories. This is because of the major active component in green tea—a chemical called EGCG. However, to garner the maximum benefit of green tea and EGCG, you must consume at least 6 to 8 cups of green tea daily, which may be difficult to do, and which even a green tea EGCG capsule won't provide. That's why NutriSystem is introducing a whole new line of green tea foods and snacks including gums, mints, and bars—all containing the important active green tea component that you can enjoy several times a day to reap the maximum benefits.

Portion Distortion

In North America, overeating has become epidemic. The number of obese people has quadrupled in the last decade, and that's taking its toll. People are dying younger, contracting more disabling diseases, and taking more medication for ailments associated with obesity. Even the number of obese children has skyrocketed almost as much as their self-esteem has plummeted. We're eating more food, more often than ever in history, and it's really starting to show.

As if the prevalence of food weren't a tough enough challenge to face, we're also constantly bombarded with portion sizes that are out of control. There is a silent crisis sweeping North America, and it's called supersizing. Supersizing is contributing to the wave of obesity that's overwhelming us.

We are getting swallowed up by the lure of "value" through brilliant marketing. We are eating far more than our healthy share of calories. We all like to get the most value for our money, but somewhere along the line we've confused supersizing with true value. Whether it's fast food, restaurant food, or the size of the cereal box you buy at the wholesale club, you need to redefine value for yourself. This is not to discourage you from making smart decisions with your shopping dollar; rather it is to encourage you to be conscious of the potential portion problems you could be buying for yourself.

In every realm, portion distortion has become an epidemic. Take the fast-food industry, for example. The average size and calorie amount of a fast-food meal has skyrocketed in the last 30 years. In 1977, the average hamburger weighed 5.7 ounces; 9 years later, it has grown to 7 ounces, and it continues to increase. Soft drinks have also grown from about 12 ounces to almost 20 ounces and larger. These increased burger and drink portions alone would cause you to gain 2 pounds a year if you ate them just once a week.

As another example of our skyrocketing portions, scientists from the University of Pennsylvania along with researchers at the Centre National de la Récherche Scientifique (CNRS) in France recently conducted a portions study. In an effort to uncover why the French population stays so slim despite all the rich cream sauces and buttery croissants they consume, researchers began studying the foods served in the cities of Philadelphia and Paris. What did they discover? They found that the average portion in Philadelphia was 25 percent larger than that in Paris, and things like chocolate bars, soft drinks, and hot dogs were up to twice the size of their counterparts in France. American yogurt was found to be a whopping 82 percent larger than the yogurt in Paris. Their overall conclusion? While what you eat matters, how much you eat can be the difference between being thin and overweight. The French paradox proves it.

It's now clear that in order to maintain a healthy weight, you must control portions and what you're consuming. Mastering the confusion around what's a true serving and how much you should be eating is one of the biggest challenges facing anyone who wants to tackle weight, but here's the good news: one of *the* best things about this program and the NutriSystem Nourish Meal Plan is that you'll always get the right amount of food for optimal weight loss—it's built right in. Doubt about serving sizes has been eliminated.

The NutriSystem Nourish program is based on appropriately sized, healthy meals. That's precisely what NutriSystem has been offering for more than 30 years—because it works. Through the program, you will learn what a true portion size is and that those portions really can satisfy you and result in effective and lasting weight loss. They're the secret to keeping the weight off for good. With the NutriSystem Nourish program, you will see your appetite rebalanced and satisfied. You'll know how much is too much.

Managing your intake has everything to do with weight loss, and even more so, your overall health. From disease prevention and longevity to weight loss and weight maintenance, keeping portions in check will do wonders for your well-being. Overeating can literally shut down your body's metabolism and fat-burning process, and consuming inflated portions will show up on your hips and thighs as well as on your cholesterol, blood sugar, and other laboratory tests.

You can control it, and through this program, you will.

Nourishment for Life

For all of us, it's all too easy to view food as something to be manipulated or cheated on to lose weight. Many of us use it as a reward or form of punishment, too. But when you shift your thinking through understanding, you begin to see food as the power you need to achieve what you hope to experience. As you learn to nourish yourself, you will learn how to satisfy and feed your true self. You will experience how to proactively and compassionately handle and heal your hunger and bring true satisfaction to your life. The way I see it, food is life giving and life affirming. Enjoy good food and you will experience a great life.

Through the NutriSystem Nourish program, you'll learn how to eat and drink the foods that support balance in your body, especially blood sugar balance (just about everything you eat and do affects this equilibrium). Here's the best news: this program's meal plan was created to provide that balance for you automatically. Through both the prepared foods and the recipes and meal plans provided, you're assured proper nutrition, including the right equilibrium of low glycemic carbs, fats, proteins and fiber. You even get the right portions—it's all built in. We've got all the nutritional bases covered for you, and that's the reason why this plan will boost your metabolism and get your body burning more fat. You won't have to worry about a thing.

What you eat serves as a building block for creating your life experience. Food is fuel, and you need to start using the ultimate grade for optimal performance.

Nourish and you'll flourish!

2

Tuning Your Metabolic Machinery

Fixing a Slow Metabolism

Have you ever felt like your metabolism was working against you? Or that it was sputtering and puttering like an old car dying for a tune-up?

I've heard my patients express this many times. Many believe that their metabolism is the reason they haven't achieved successful weight loss. Take Susan, for example.

> Susan, age 46, had been a serial dieter for most of her adult life. She was convinced when she came in to see me that her ability to lose weight was lost due to what she called her "slow, barely breathing metabolism." Susan tried to convince me that she either was going to have to give up on her metabolism altogether or become a marathon runner to revive her ability to burn. When I discussed the right way to lose weight with her, she questioned me with disbelief but agreed to try it. Susan had always complained of having cold feet and hands, but in 2 weeks, she noticed that her circulation seemed to improve, as did her ability to move without pain and strain. After 1 month, Susan was sleeping better, her cravings for sugar and salt were no longer an issue, and she had lost 16 pounds!

The plan had kicked in her metabolism and I never heard Susan complain about it again.

I tell my patients this all the time, but it's so true: your metabolism is not trying to conspire against you. It's quite the opposite. Your body has an infinite wisdom—trust it! It was built to serve you. When you overly limit food intake or skip meals, your body will probably move into storage mode. But if you feed it well and at regular intervals, it will respond by burning the fuel with metabolic excellence.

Your metabolism has a profound effect on how much weight you will lose over a period of time, so in order to lose weight, you need to maximize your metabolism—and on the NutriSystem Nourish program, you will become a powerful, fat-burning machine in no time.

Maybe you've tried many different diets, which probably means that your metabolism may be in need of repair, especially if you've been on any of the extremely low-calorie diets that often lead to a quick return to your original weight and then some. Soon after the diet begins, you experience a calorie debt that prompts your metabolism to slow down in an effort to conserve and preserve energy and life. Your body thinks it's starving, and it does everything it can to conserve fat for survival. Your metabolism is then further disturbed when you eventually decide to quit that low-calorie program and resume a reasonable calorie plan, which requires your metabolism to adapt once again.

If you've been on these diets and your weight is constantly going up and down, your metabolism has likely slowed down, and I'm sure it has become harder and harder for you to lose weight. But don't despair! This program understands all that, and it was designed specifically to help you reconfigure your metabolism and get your body burning fat again.

Time for a Tune-Up?

If you answer yes to any of these questions, it may be time for a metabolic tune-up:

- *Scarcity:* Have you ever been on a starvation diet that only left you feeling deprived and struggling to lose weight?
- *Bingeing:* Are you experienced with diets on which you were starving all day and eating all night?
- *Low energy:* Have you ever taken part in a dieting plan that left you looking at the morning alarm clock as if it were a personal attack on you?
- *Moodiness:* Do you ever overreact—like getting mad at traffic signals or yelling at your family when dialogue would do?

The NutriSystem Nourish Fat-Burning Principles

Metabolism is all about continually fueling your body so that it's constantly burning fat. That's exactly what this program was designed to do. By following the NutriSystem Nourish program, you can put an end to any roller coaster weight effect you may have experienced through other diets and instead fine-tune your metabolic machine for top performance. The whole point of this program is to rev up your metabolism so that your body burns more fat—and it's not that difficult to do. You simply need to focus on four main things. I refer to these as the NutriSystem Nourish Fat-Burning Principles:

1. *Eat well.* We just learned about nutrition and using food as fuel in Chapter One. By eating foods with low glycemic values and optimal levels of proteins and healthy fats, you will balance your blood sugar levels, encourage a healthy hormonal chemistry, and keep your metabolism burning well.

2. *Eat often.* As important to your metabolism as what you eat is how often you eat. The key is to eat five times a day: breakfast, lunch, dinner, and two snacks. Small, frequent meals and healthy snacks foster more constant blood sugar levels and keep your metabolism at peak performance throughout the day so that you can burn fat nonstop.

3. *Exercise.* Exercise is a key ingredient to metabolic excellence. Little movement, little burn. When we talk about exercise in Chapter Six, you'll see that even a little extra movement can make a big difference in how your metabolism performs for you. If you dread exercise now, you'll change and begin to see it as one of your greatest allies.

4. *Minimize stress.* This is extremely key to your metabolism, too. In Chapter Four you'll find out exactly why, but for now, know that how you deal with stress and how you release it will have a huge impact on what you weigh and your overall health.

The NutriSystem Nourish program was built on these four fat-burning principles. Everything—from the foods you eat and how often you eat them to the exercises you do and the mindset you create for yourself—centers around these principles and works to turn your body into a fat-burning machine.

By embracing the NutriSystem Nourish fat-burning principles and putting them into action every day, you will be managing not only your metabolism but also your entire hormonal chemistry.

A Day in the Life of NutriSystem Nourish

Peggy combines the Prepared Foods Meal Plan and the Do-It-Yourself Meal Plan for her weight-loss program.

Peggy is a busy mom with two teenage sons and 75 pounds to lose. It's Saturday, and her schedule is packed. Knowing this, she set her alarm a half-hour early the night before to make sure to fit in some personal care time for herself first thing in the morning. She wakes and does a morning "Bookend Routine" before heading into the kitchen to whip up a Cheese Omelet (from the NutriSystem Nourish recipes). Along with some strawberries it's a great start to a big day.

Peggy packs a quick lunch to take with her and heads out the door to her son's morning football game. She spends the first two quarters watching the game from the stadium's track, where she's walking some laps, and by halftime she's in the stands enjoying her NutriSystem Pasta Salad with Ham, some celery sticks, and a bag of NutriSystem White Cheddar Soy Chips.

After the game (they won!) she stops by the mall with her boys to pick up a birthday gift for her sister, and on the way she munches on the apple she had thrown in her purse. After a few more errands, she's back home and ready for an enjoyable evening. She fixes Chicken Cacciatore (another NutriSystem Nourish recipe) for herself and the kids, then they all head out to the latest movie. Along with her NutriSystem Chocolate Peanut Butter Dessert Bar, it's a pretty good show. Peggy completes the day with an evening "Bookend Routine" and looks forward to Sunday.

It's been another great day on the NutriSystem Nourish program for Peggy.

Hormonal Excellence

Optimal metabolism begins and ends with hormonal excellence. Have you ever heard yourself say, "It's not me, it's my hormones," or, "It's not me, it's my metabolism"? There is a good chance you were right, especially when it comes to weight gain and how you burn fat. Hormones play a role in every physiological process in your body, including how well your metabolism works. Hormones are always trying to maintain balance and harmony in your system—that's their job.

Knowing how to use food as a powerful activator to support your hormones is key to supporting robust metabolism and optimal weight loss, and it's something you'll be doing automatically by following the NutriSystem Nourish plan. The basic fat-burning principles—eating well, eating often, exercising, and minimizing stress—help to maintain a steady hormonal balance, which in turn strengthens your metabolism even more. They're all interlinked. Your body is designed to respond to the foods you eat and create a hormonal response to meet its needs, much like the workings of a finely tuned machine. Knowing this, through good eating habits and a well-rounded approach to weight loss, you can empower yourself and your body chemistry to become a fat-burning metabolic miracle.

> ### Your Choices, Your Metabolism
>
> Consider this: After you eat a meal containing a large amount of carbohydrates or fat, your metabolic rate usually increases about 4 percent. By contrast, after you consume a meal containing optimal amounts of protein and low-glycemic carbohydrates, your metabolic rate usually begins to increase within 1 hour, reaches a maximum of about 30 percent above normal, and stays there, burning, as long as 3 to 12 hours.
>
> You can control your metabolism and burn more fat if you nourish yourself well every day.

Timing Is Everything

Your eating schedule is crucial when it comes to increasing your metabolism, and it all has to do with preventing a state of low blood sugar. This happens after a high-glycemic carbohydrate meal is eaten, causing blood sugar levels to first rise, then decline too quickly. As you know, this is caused by an excess of insulin being released and too much sugar is drawn out of the blood, which then causes blood sugar levels to fall below normal and causes fat to be stored. Symptoms of low blood sugar include uncontrollable hunger, moodiness, anxiety, shakiness, perspiration, lack of energy, mental confusion, anger, and more. This continuous state can also be a forerunner to type 2 diabetes, a disease that often goes hand-in-hand with obesity.

The secret to avoiding low blood sugar lies in eating nourishing foods, including low-glycemic carbohydrates, every 3 to 4 hours, and that's what the NutriSystem Nourish program recommends. When you come to the meal plan section of this book, you'll see that we've outlined some specific meal plans for you to follow, all of which ensure that your body gets fed frequently to keep your metabolism going.

When you're on the NutriSystem Nourish program, there are two ways you can go when it comes to managing your meal plan. The first meal plan option you have is to prepare all of the foods on the NutriSystem Nourish plan on your own, buying as many whole foods as possible and preparing everything as fresh as possible. You'll be cooking up healthy dishes and can rely on many of the recipes in this book to ensure a healthy, balanced diet. For those of you able and willing to do this, I say go for it. Your body, your mind, and your metabolism will thank you for the fresh, wholesome foods.

But let's face it—many of us are just too busy to prepare five healthy meals a day. Finding the time, let alone the energy, to do all that is a challenge and you might not eat on time. This program has a solution for you, too.

If you lead a busy lifestyle and have a million and one things to do every day, don't despair. You can still get the great balance of healthy, low-glycemic foods about every few hours with NutriSystem's new, ready-to-go prepared foods. You can get everything from breakfasts to lunch and dinner entrees— even great-tasting snacks and desserts to fill in the gaps—and it's all healthy, balanced, and immediately ready to go. It's all portable, so you can take your meals with you wherever you go, and there are almost a hundred different meals and desserts available (see a complete listing of the new NutriSystem Nourish foods in Chapter 5). All are based on a low-glycemic index and offer optimal levels of protein and fats to help your body burn fat best. You simply combine them with fresh fruits and vegetables and your plan is ready to go.

For years thousands of people have had success eating NutriSystem's prepared meals, because along with tasting great, they do one other thing very well—they keep you prepared. NutriSystem truly takes the work out of weight loss. They do all the prep work, all the calorie counting, glycemic-index measuring, and portion control for you. All you need to do is remember to eat every few hours, and bam—you kick your metabolism into high gear.

Or you can do a combination meal plan, preparing some meals yourself and eating NutriSystem's prepared meals at other times when you're busy. The choice is up to you.

But whichever meal plan you utilize—cooking whole foods on your own based on the NutriSystem Nourish meal plan, or buying the Nutri-System Nourish prepared foods—by eating every few hours, you'll avoid low blood sugar levels and hunger and you'll keep your metabolism burning strong.

The Snack Is Back!

Now you know why it's imperative that you eat something about every 3 to 4 hours—because the strength of your metabolism depends on it—but does that mean you're supposed to be eating big, full meals that often?

Not exactly. On the NutriSystem Nourish program, our meal plan features three meals (breakfast, lunch, and dinner), but it also includes two healthy snacks every day. In total, you'll be eating five times a day, fueling your body with healthy carbs, proteins, and fats to maximize your metabolism, which means the snack is back.

Many diets discourage snacking but not this one. We meet the age-old "To snack or not to snack?" question with a resounding yes because we know that healthy snacking can be key to revving up that metabolism of yours. However, before you start munching, it's a good idea to consider the fact that often the majority of our snacking is due to something other than hunger. We're all human, and we're all affected by myriad things in our lives. Stress, loneliness, boredom, or even feelings of celebration can often be the main impetus behind an urge to snack. So when you initially feel the desire to snack, stop for a moment and ask yourself, "Do I really need to eat, or is something eating at me?" Be honest. When you really think about why you want a snack, if you find a cause other than true hunger that's making you want to munch (like the fact that your sister or husband or mother will never understand, or your boss couldn't care less), that's okay. Just don't go for food in that instance; it will never satisfy you. Instead, search for a different, healthier alternative to snacking. Release the emotion you may be feeling instead of letting it lead you to some snack food.

That said, if you're dying for a snack and true hunger is what you are really experiencing, let the snacking begin. Strategic snacking, as scheduled in the meal plans, can do wonders for balance and optimum wellness. It can increase alertness, energy, productivity, metabolism, and optimism, and it can help you to manage and lose weight. Just remember, when it comes to snacking, there are two important elements: type and timing.

For starters, you need to know what types of snacks deliver the best outcome and the most satisfaction. They must be slow burning, blood sugar balancing, and energy sustaining—for example, cottage cheese, nuts, seeds, apples, pears, and yogurt. If you're using the NutriSystem Nourish foods, you'll even get soy chips and high-protein chocolate.

Next, you must consider the proper timing of your snacks. On the NutriSystem Nourish meal plan, you're scheduled to eat three meals a day and two healthy snacks to keep your body burning. Say you're hungry, but your next meal is more than 2 hours away; your blood sugar is fading, and your irritability is rising. What should you do? In this instance, it's wise to choose a snack for greater sustenance, such as fruits like apples and celery with 2 tablespoons of a nut (or seed) butter spread on top, or a protein-enriched soy and fruit smoothie.

Of course, it all depends on what you've chosen to stock your kitchen with, but the main message when it comes to snacking is to do so sensibly and strategically. Always remember: *type and timing*. Whenever possible, plan ahead to avoid getting caught with your blood sugar down and no good choices around. Do all you can to avoid the quick-fix, empty calorie, sugary snacks like soda and candy bars. Although they'll lift you quickly, they'll drop you even faster and they will just leave you hungry for more. They'll spike your insulin every time, and as you know, that pretty much means metabolism breakdown and fat storage.

Stress and Your Metabolism

Stress has a very detrimental effect on metabolism. Like skipping meals and making poor meal and snack choices, stress can wreak havoc on your metabolism but in a slightly different way. Being continuously overstressed leads to muscle loss, and muscle loss leads to a decrease in metabolic rate, making it more difficult to burn calories. In a nutshell, ongoing stress leads to a hormone imbalance that decreases muscle and its ability to help you burn fat.

If that isn't enough to get you to take that vacation in Tahiti, I don't know what is. Just think—the more you'd relax on the beach, the more efficiently your metabolism would burn, and you'd look that much better in your swimsuit! I address the effect of stress on weight gain and weight loss much more extensively in Chapter Four, but know that managing stress, and living a balanced, centered life is key to long-term weight-loss success.

Vicious Cycles

What happens if you fall short? What happens when you skip breakfast and it's 3 P.M. before you realize that you haven't had anything except 4 cups of coffee all day? What if the last time you exercised was in 1982? Whatever the cause, what's the effect? The biggest problem with any of those metabolism busters is that they lead to more metabolism busting.

Say, for instance, you miss your eating windows quite often. You skip meals here and there, and are just too busy to grab a snack between lunch and dinner. This sets your metabolism up for a lot of challenges. Most significantly, your blood sugar level is challenged and your insulin level fluctuates, while your body is asked to perform without the right fuel. In a reactive state, your body begins replacing muscle tissue with fat, and this directly affects your metabolism (because muscle is what helps the body burn fat). Once you go into this state, you're losing muscle, which means you're losing some ability to burn fat. So skipping meals is not helping you lose weight.

Five Reasons Why Starvation and Deprivation Don't Work

1. Your body has a powerful will to survive, and if you miss or skip meals, your body sees this as a threat to its survival and it has one choice—to stop burning and start storing fat.

2. Your mind and your brain need a constant fuel supply to give you a feeling of confidence and satisfaction. If you block that fuel source, get ready to watch your cravings take over.

3. When your body is not given enough to live on—when you skip meals or avoid food altogether—it is forced to use your muscle tissue for food. When you lose muscle, you lose metabolism!

4. Food is energy. In order to move well, you need to eat well and eat frequently. If you miss meals, you'll lose the ability to move, and if you stop moving, you'll stop burning.

5. You are the beauty of mind, body, and soul. Starving your body serves only to deprive your entire self. Metabolism is more than just fat burning—it is your energy and passion for life. Eating with purpose fuels a life full of passion!

As another example, take a situation where someone is eating quite often and snacking quite regularly, but his or her choices lack merit. In other words, a guy is hitting the vending machine every hour and a half (I think everybody knows someone like that). While he's certainly doing his best to fuel his body often, his poor choices are killing his metabolism.

To thrive, your brain needs to have its share of its favorite fuel source: sugar. It's not only your taste buds that crave that giant chocolate bar! When you eat out of balance or eat high-glycemic carbohydrates, you set yourself up for a blood sugar roller coaster just like when you skip meals, which only increases your cravings for more sugar. Your body starts to crave sugar, so you grab a sugary or high-carb snack, which immediately translates into a lot of sugar in your body. That makes your insulin surge and blood sugar levels spike but then shortly thereafter crash. Your brain experiences that dip in blood sugar and translates it into the need to get even more sweets, fast. So you crave again and head back to the vendo-land for another big bag of candy. Not only have you sabotaged your metabolism, but with this pattern you will most likely experience moodiness, irritability, and anxiousness.

> **Nourishing Moment**
>
> Sometimes managing your weight is all about your attitude and approach toward food. The next time you head into the kitchen, notice your body language as you approach your refrigerator, pantry, or cupboard. If you are experiencing a sense of disempowerment and vulnerability, simply adjust your posture to reflect confidence and courageous conviction. Lift your head, adjust your shoulders, breathe deeply, and envision the outcome you desire. Amazingly, you'll make better choices!

The solution in both instances, whether you're not eating frequently enough or not eating well enough, is to feed your body more regularly with better food, or risk the blood sugar roller coaster and all its ripple effects. These choices are in your hands, and once you understand what's going on in your body after you eat something, you can choose wisely and choose your own metabolism.

Choose Your Own Metabolism

You truly can choose your own metabolism. Managing the way your body burns fat and achieving success on this program are all within your control, whether you realize it or not. It's something you'll experience very soon, and when you do, you'll be amazed how it changes your life.

Weight-loss success is all about choices and learning what it takes to make good ones. By following the NutriSystem Nourish program, you'll learn to choose foods with the end in mind. And while that may sound a bit esoteric or out there to you, it's a very real outcome when you follow the NutriSystem Nourish program.

We all have an idea in mind of how we'd like to feel after a meal. How do you want to feel after you eat? Energized or ready for a nap? How do you wish to feel emotionally after you eat? Inspired or remorseful? You need to create a clear objective in your mind each time before you eat. You need to set a goal as to how you want your eating experience to end.

Perhaps you're a bowler. If so, envision the end of your meal as one big strike zone, with all 10 pins standing staunch in the center. When you're finished eating, how will you have scored? Did you get the strike you were aiming for or was your meal a gutter ball? If you think about where you're going before you begin, you're much more likely to get there. This mentality applies whether you're talking about one meal or one lifetime. If you can't see your strike zone, then it's pretty doubtful you'll get many pins down.

You need to find an eating plan that supports your goals. This program does that because it was designed with the knowledge that a goal is far different from any quick fix. When you're surrounded by the number of eating choices that we all have these days, you need a balanced plan for success. When your hormones are in balance, your body is in balance and your metabolism soars.

My patients have repeatedly told me that on this low-glycemic program their previously insatiable sugar cravings gave way to a sense of control with little to no cravings at all. When you follow the NutriSystem Nourish program and eat in balance, your body chemistry will move to its normal healthy rhythm and you will get those same results. You will feel more satisfied, you will crave less, and you will desire to eat less. Your energy will improve, your mood will be positive, and your whole self will be empowered. All of the energy you used to fight fatigue, sugar cravings, hunger, and hormone imbalances will now be channeled toward building and enjoying your life. Now that's a score.

You may have the best of intentions, but let's face it—sometimes it's easier to give in to cravings and short-term satisfaction, which only lead to more binge eating, more weight gain, and a whole lot of guilt and

Metabolic Minutes

Here are five quick things you can do during your day to jumpstart your metabolism in no time.

1. *Kitchen curls.* While waiting for water to boil or the buzzer to go off on the stove or microwave, grab a couple of soup cans and do 20 bicep curls and shoulder lifts. Repeat this 3 times.

2. *The no-rest room.* While brushing your teeth, do a series of modified squats by standing in front of the toilet (lid down) and sitting so that your bottom barely and briefly touches the seat of your toilet. Stand and repeat 15 times.

3. *Television tummy buffers.* When you're watching TV or during commercial breaks, try these metabolism boosters:
   - Walk or dance in place.
   - Do one set of 12 modified push-ups.
   - Do one set of 12 modified lunges on each side.
   - Sit on an exercise ball rather than lounging on the sofa.

4. *Meeting movements.* During a meeting or when you're in your car or at your desk, practice conscious breathing from your belly while also flexing and releasing each muscle group: buttocks, thighs, stomach, arms. Repeat this as often as possible.

5. *Take a lap.* Before you enter your house, kitchen, cafeteria, or even just a restaurant, take a lap around the yard, hallway, parking lot, or neighborhood.

depressing fault finding afterward. But while good choices can be tough to make, with the backing of a program like NutriSystem Nourish, you can and will make them, because you'll be balanced, in control, and free to focus on your goal.

Plan to Succeed

When it comes to losing weight and keeping your metabolism fueled, once you have your goals in mind, you just need to be prepared. That way, you can stop any problems or negative behavior before they even start.

My wife and I try to plan meals ahead of time on the weekend for the following week and we do a big grocery shopping trip so that we can look forward to a whole week of healthful eating. Once we're home, we immediately prewash, dry, and chop at least half of the vegetables we've bought, then store them in zipper bags in the refrigerator. That way, they're readily accessible morning, noon, and night—and so are the good choices. Having everything that you need on hand is extremely key.

I'm certain you, too, have had to prepare for something, whether it be a test in school, a job interview, an athletic event, the birth of a child, or just simply getting set for a day in your life. And I'm sure you realized that the quality of your preparation was a powerful catalyst for both your confidence and your success.

Now think of a time when you may have been on a diet plan and you had the best of intentions to stay with it and get the results you envisioned, but then life kind of happened and got in the way of your plans. It could have been that you were so busy running around that by default you had to make less-than-desirable choices because there was nothing else available at the time. Or perhaps you were at work or driving the kids to soccer practice all day and you hadn't found the time to put something together the night before, so there you were . . . stressed, hungry, and vulnerable . . . and forced to do whatever you could to get through the day, like going to the drive-through, the vending machine, or eating nothing at all. All these scenarios are very real. They can be a real challenge to your weight-loss commitment not to mention a major problem as they throw your metabolism into a state of flux.

But remember, you can control all of this.

By planning ahead, you plan for success. Give yourself a leg up by finding ways to remind yourself to eat. If you're at work, place reminders around your desk to eat at regular intervals. Use sticky notes, chalkboards, or even the clock on your computer to remind you to eat and fuel your mind. Or if you're out and about, set your watch to beep when you're supposed to eat or ask your best friend or someone you trust to call you at a certain time. Not only will your metabolism thank you but you'll also be continually reminded of your commitment and desire to succeed.

It's all about routine and a little bit of planning. Do it and you'll see results. I've seen it with my patients, and it's something the folks at Nutri-System have known for years. Those who prepare for success succeed. Based on that knowledge, we created this program with built-in quick and easy solutions for keeping you on track. All you need is the intention and the desire to make it happen and the program will support you in actualizing your vision. Guaranteed!

Burn, Baby, Burn

When it comes to metabolism, it's a pretty straightforward deal. You need to eat well, eat often, exercise, and minimize stress. You also need to make good choices, one after another, and to make sure you're always prepared for success.

The good news is that your body is designed to be metabolically efficient. It's a fat-burning machine and you have control over its efficiency. Sure, we're all given a little different body chemistry. And sure, hormones and even your age factor into your body's fat-burning process. But with a little know-how and some fine-tuning of your routine you can have your metabolism up and running at top speed in no time.

3

Mind Over Matter

Losing Weight Without
Losing Your Mind

Think of a time when you were at peace with yourself—when you were truly at peace with both your body and your mind. A time when all things were working in harmony and you didn't strain to find energy. Your mind was clear and alert.

Think back to a time when you didn't worry about how your body looked and your mind was calm. Maybe it was when you were a kid. Maybe it was that summer when you toured the country. Maybe it was that day when you just couldn't stop smiling.

That kind of clarity, that place of peace, is actually your natural state of being. And it comes from being well nourished both in body and mind.

We've just spent the last two chapters talking about how to use food as fuel and how to harness the various ways of fine-tuning your body mechanics. The key to any weight-loss plan is mastery over nutrition and how you use food to get your body going. But an equally important force in the success of any weight-loss or life plan is the mind. What goes into it and certainly what comes out of it are the catalyst for everything. What many people (and many weight-loss plans, for that matter) tend to forget is that the mind plays a crucial role in shaping the body. Even if you do everything to make your body a well-oiled machine, it truly won't go anywhere without its driver—the mind.

Your mind can be a powerful force in weight-loss success and life transformation.

41

The NutriSystem Nourish program acknowledges this important fact. It takes into account not only what's going on physically inside your body but also what's going on inside your head, and how your mindset and lifestyle patterns affect your weight-loss efforts. This is a crucial element to the weight-loss process. The mind matters.

As we go through this chapter, I'm going to ask you to take a mental inventory of your thoughts and your thinking patterns.

- Are you a priority in your own life?
- What beliefs do you carry with you about yourself?
- Does your current thinking inspire you or do you have a foreboding outlook?

I'm also going to ask you to notice what's surrounding you in your life. Even if you don't realize it, much of what you think about is coming or growing directly out of what's around you. Have you ever spent time with a friend who is a downer? How do you feel after an evening with a pessimist? Are you inspired or depressed after watching the news? In contrast, how do you feel when you see or do something you love—say going to a favorite concert or joining in to help with a pet project? How does your favorite photo make you feel? The things around us, the things we expose ourselves to every day, affect our mind, and our mind affects our body. Once you have learned how to harness the power of all that, you'll have unbounded power to shape the rest of your life.

The NutriSystem Nourish program will help you cultivate the life you desire. To do it, you must nourish both your body and mind well by allowing the process to unfold and to reinvent yourself, reshaping your experience of life. Your body will begin working for you, and by shaping up your mind, you'll start overcoming the mental obstacles that are inhibiting your weight loss. Just open yourself up to the idea and give yourself permission to nourish yourself without expectation.

In my first appointment with Dr. James, I asked him to just give me a diet and tell me how much weight I needed to lose. But as I tried to lose weight, something just was not coming together. I was feeling at odds with my commitment, and on a deeper level, I was truly struggling with my faith in myself to follow through on something that was just for me. I felt that I was experiencing my life in two separate places: one was the body trying to lose weight, eat better, move more; the other me was stuck in the "you cannot stay with this—

who are you kidding?" mode. But as I worked on the daily practices that Dr. James outlined for me, I felt that for the first time in my life I could count on me—the whole me—to step up and take a stand to become a better, more whole person, and I'm now at my desired weight!—Tina, age 42

A Day in the Life of NutriSystem Nourish

Charlie and Diane follow the Do-It-Yourself Meal Plan 100 percent for their weight-loss program.

Charlie and Diane moved to Vermont two years ago, and while endeavoring to lose weight, they are thoroughly enjoying living healthy and fit in their retirement. It's Friday, and they awake slowly to enjoy some light vanilla yogurt and a Banana Chocolate Chip Muffin over coffee and the daily crossword puzzle. Once fully awake, they head out for a walk down their lane, taking turns doing their "mental floss" exercise out loud, dispelling some negative thoughts and sharing more positive ones together. By lunchtime, they're keeping their weekly volunteer date at the local hospital and stop by the cafeteria for a grilled chicken salad, some low-salt rye crackers, and a big glass of milk. Once home, it's almost 3 P.M., and they grab a handful of raisins and a slice of fat-free cheese while working through some bills and receipts.

For dinner, Tilapia with Honey Mustard Sauce (from the NutriSystem Nourish recipes) is on the menu, and Diane fits in a few "Metabolic Minutes"—doing a few sets of arm curls with a can of soup—while waiting for the fish fillets to broil. After chatting on the phone with the grandkids after supper, they both relax with a piece of homemade Creamy Baked Cheesecake with Blueberry Topping (another Nutri-System Nourish recipe) while watching *Law & Order* on TV.

It's been another great day on the NutriSystem Nourish program for Charlie and Diane.

Becoming who you want to be involves creating a positive, healthy relationship with your body and mind. We're drawn to that and to people who have achieved that. Over the years, I've identified five basic things people do with their mindset to foster this healthy relationship. Doing these things can help you focus your mind and get your attitude in gear. You need to:

1. Prioritize yourself.
2. Examine your beliefs.

3. Use your "mental floss."
4. Create a positive mindset.
5. Set new goals.

In this chapter, I'm going to walk you through each of these elements and give you exercises to practice that can help you accomplish these five things. Once you provide yourself with concrete food for thought, you will notice how your hunger, needs, and desires begin to shift. Think about it: How often do you make your way to the kitchen to satisfy your latest desire when you are really hungering for something deeper? How often do you search outside of yourself for solutions to challenges in your life? By balancing your mind, you'll gain new perspective and begin to nourish your entire life from the inside out. If you can restructure your mindset, you can start to see new and different ways of living and being.

1. Prioritize Yourself

You probably don't often say, "Gosh, I just have so much time on my hands and nothing to do." Most people who I see seem to be collectively suffering from the epidemic I call chronic "overdoingitis."

I see many people who are working on weight issues who have found themselves fairly far down the list when it comes to taking care of themselves. And yes, to be open and willing to making yourself a greater priority can be scary and quite uncomfortable. I can already hear you engaging in the inner dialogue of "That would be selfish of me" or "I cannot think of such a thing," but you need to be clear with the truth that self-love and self-care are not self-indulgent. I know it may be difficult to find the time for yourself, especially if you have children and/or a hectic career, but you must gain your own balance and be able to really focus on your goal of losing weight to be successful.

Let me emphasize that again for importance: *loving yourself and caring for yourself do not mean you're being self-indulgent.* In fact, doing so is a prerequisite for moving ahead and graduating into a life experience of joy, peace, and fulfillment. Otherwise, you'll never make the grade.

To successfully lose weight, you need to begin to view both you and your weight-loss goal as priorities. This cannot be done just in thought or philosophy, either. It must also become evident in action. And to do so, you can begin with your typical list-making duties—you know, the big list you sit down to write however many times a week that says "to do" at the top. First, I want you to do this: rename that list your "TO YOU" list. (Just by doing that, you're already on the right track!) Next, as you are jotting down all your daily or weekly tasks, take a good look at what's there. Where are *you* on that list? Do you rank up high or lower down the line? Are you lost among the shopping, the soccer practice, the career, or the laundry? Are you even on the list at all?

Clinically and personally, I have seen time and time again that those people who are courageous enough to see themselves at the top of their own to-do list have the most success losing weight. It's a common thread. They prioritize their walk, their food prep, their personal downtime, or whatever else makes their program work for them above all other tasks of daily living. I also know that doing that isn't easy for them; in fact, when most began doing it, it was pretty uncomfortable for them.

Your To-You List

Take a moment to notice where *you* are on your daily to-do list. Begin today to move yourself to the top of your list by:

- Taking a walk or doing your exercise first thing in the morning
- Stopping by the grocery store before you run out of fresh food
- Making an appointment and keeping it for a massage, pedicure, or haircut
- Scheduling a wellness or mental health day
- Saying no when asked to do too much
- Organizing your meal plan and foods for the coming day
- Stopping to take deep breaths throughout your day
- Buying a new book and reading it
- Ending the day with a bath with real lavender oil in it

Most people, particularly women, are downright embarrassed or ashamed to put themselves first. How we got to this place, I'm not sure, but I know we need to leave it. Any of you who spend time with children know that we certainly weren't born this way. When we come into this world, we believe the world revolves around us for at least the first 10 years of life. There's a reason why *mine!* is one of the first words we say. But as I've watched my patients work at putting themselves first, I've seen such interesting things begin to happen for them. Their energy shifts and they come alive with purpose, and many find that they actually get a lot more done on a day-to-day basis once they've made themselves a priority.

In order to lose weight and improve your fitness and health, you must decide to nourish and *value* yourself first. These days, that may mean unlearning the popular programming that you are not enough. You *are* enough just as you are, and there's no reason to beat yourself up about anything. Sure, life sometimes takes you away from your true self; you get caught up in all that you're doing and get too busy, too afraid, or just feel downright powerless to change your ways. But through the NutriSystem Nourish program, you can regain control. Success can happen for you, too, if you simply take time to value yourself. Here's how.

Start by doing this: Pick a weekend afternoon and take time to sit down and plan out the week ahead. Make at least two walking dates with friends, set aside time for journaling, and plan nightly rituals such as taking a bath with essential oils. Schedule in things you like to do that are good for you. This is an opportunity to follow through and support your new belief systems, so don't waste it. Then throughout the following week, follow through on all those plans you outlined. At first it won't be easy to keep those commitments and it may be difficult to change too much overnight. But slowly you will see your perception of your own worth increase and the uncomfortable nature of taking time for yourself decrease in the wake of great joy, fulfillment, and purpose.

Don't just trust me on this—try it for yourself!

Once you start truly making yourself a priority, you will start to find time that you thought you never had before, and you'll continually gain clarity about that which you no longer value—you'll be able to let those things go. Intentionally put yourself at the top of your to-you list and be clear about who you are and where you want to go. Remember, you are the one who can create and experience all that you desire—one step, one list, one nourishing gesture to yourself at a time.

2. Examine Your Beliefs

Once you've learned to view yourself compassionately as a priority, it's time to evaluate those things that you truly believe about yourself. It has been said that if you want to know the state of your belief system, just

Soft Eyes

Making yourself a priority involves treating yourself with compassion. Instead of judging yourself critically, begin seeing yourself and others more kindly and try to be more loving, accepting, and encouraging.

There's a "soft eyes" practice I learned while spending time in India and Nepal. A meditation instructor encouraged me to consider how often we tend to look at others critically and judgmentally. He referred to that pattern and condition as looking at the world with "hard eyes." He then asked me to think about how often we look at ourselves with hard eyes that are judgmental and often hurtful.

Then he instructed me to open to the practice of seeing others and myself with "soft eyes." Soft eyes are loving, accepting, and encouraging. Soft eyes are open with love and reflect an open, loving heart. Viewing the world through soft eyes can make a profound difference in how you approach life and your weight-loss effort. You'll develop a confidence and trust in yourself that will help you stay on track and support your goals every day. Say kind things to yourself. Instead of cutting yourself down, start seeing things through soft eyes. By applying this practice through-out your daily life, you'll see how it changes your life.

I remember the first time Dr. James talked to me about the soft eyes practice. I wanted to laugh in his face and say something like, "That's the lamest advice I've ever heard." But then the next day I noticed that I kept thinking more about it and just for kicks I decided to give it a try. I was amazed at how I had been judging everybody, including myself, and everything, and how that line between my eyes was probably a manifestation of my critical outlook on life. I was horrified to notice that I had been using hard eyes around my children, my husband, and most of my friends. I certainly had hard eyes at the grocery store and when I looked in the mirror each morning. I also had hard eyes when it came to my own self-judgment about my weight. Needless to say, the soft eyes practice didn't come easily for me. I keep a journal of my feelings and just keep trying to soften my gaze and focus on loving kindness. What happened after about a week is that my friends and family first thought that I was a little crazy, but then they shared that I seemed like a new person, a more joyous person. The funny thing is, I never knew that I wasn't that person before. This process helped me get my priorities back on track and helped me lose weight in the process.—Patricia, 48 look around you and you'll see that which you believe in. Or, at least it's a start.

Getting clear about your beliefs is an important step in creating a breakthrough in weight loss. In my clinic, I see daily how people's beliefs serve as the foundation for their success or failure, especially when it comes to reaching a weight-loss goal.

Ask yourself these questions:

- Do I believe I can be successful with losing and then maintaining my ideal healthy weight?
- What beliefs do I have about myself when it comes to food, dieting, and my self-care?
- Do I believe that I have the ability and conviction to do what I know in my heart to be true to transform the quality of my life and become the person of my dreams?

Unless you decide to take a look and truly examine your beliefs, you are most likely going to recreate the same old patterns and behaviors in your life. For example, you may believe that sugar has some power over you. You're always giving in to your craving for it, yet you want to change that behavior. How do you think that inner belief about sugar is going to affect your efforts? Doesn't it leave you feeling fairly powerless? Doesn't that belief translate into a long-term relationship with sugar that is less than inspiring?

When we believe something, we behave in a way that plays out that belief, even if the belief is something we do not want to experience. You behave based on your beliefs whether you like it or not. So if you want to change a behavior—to transform a relationship with food, exercise, or life—you need to change your belief about it first.

Your beliefs are a window to your world and shape your experience either positively or negatively. They act as a filter for the world around you. Everything is affected either positively or negatively through your beliefs. When it comes to diet programs, you may believe that all programs are destined to eventually fail you, or that you will eventually fail on the program.

Instead, be open to new beliefs about yourself and your ability to succeed.

The NutriSystem Nourish program is integrated so that you are able to bring the power of your mind to the goal of weight loss. Your mind and your beliefs about yourself are going to be the difference in your truly experiencing long-term success and life fulfillment.

Think about the fact that if you are doing just a diet and you're not dealing with your belief system, then when you reach your goal of X amount of pounds lost, you still will not have changed your lifestyle and you will not see yourself as someone who has truly created change. Will you experience long-term success, peace, and happiness with this approach? Not a chance.

Nourish new beliefs and you can change your life.

But through our program, you have the opportunity to transform your body, your mind, and your life—together at once. With a little faith in yourself, together with the NutriSystem Nourish program backing you up, you can reshape your mind so that it can take you and your body anywhere you want to go.

3. Use Your "Mental Floss"

Most of our thoughts are recycled. That's good news if you are one of the few positive and optimistic thinkers around. However, that's not-so-good news if you are among the majority of folks who tend toward limited and small thinking. Even if you don't mean to be pessimistic, if what's running through your head is anything less than encouraging, you're constantly hearing negative ideas and opinions, and trust me, you're listening.

Some of us have more baggage than others and some of us struggle to envision new ways. But in one way or another, if you're going to succeed with weight loss and changing your destructive patterns for good, you need to clear out the bad stuff in your mind and start anew. In the same way you established previous patterns of thinking, you now need to create new ones. Those negative messages didn't arrive there overnight. It took time and cultivation for them to grow strong. And of all the emotions that we can experience, there's not one more damaging and paralyzing to weight-loss success than guilt or shame. The negativity they cause can be enough to keep hope at bay, and you from realizing your true potential. What good could they ever offer you?

To succeed, you need to let go of any old, haunting beliefs about yourself. If you're courageous and face those things that bring you down, you can bring the healing emotions of compassion and acceptance into this process now. Compassion and acceptance of *you*—you and all of your humanness, your beauty and awkwardness, your failures and successes, and your life lived up to now—can be gained through your new soft and accepting eyes.

If you are open and willing to heal, you can let go of any history that no longer supports or aligns with who you are today and that better place where you are definitely headed.

"But" Reduction Exercise

Many times in our lives, our *buts* get in our way:

- But I've just always been this way.
- But I've never been successful.
- But who's going to help me?
- But why am I always the one feeling this way?

Our lists can go on and on, and often we don't even realize how many times we *but* our way right out of our own potential. But not anymore! This simple exercise is an opportunity to identify all of the buts in your life that you would like to get rid of. It's a chance to realize how often you make excuses and to make a positive shift in your life.

Sit down and take inventory of any beliefs about yourself or any worn-out stories that you know are not supporting you now and where you want to be going. Write each of them down specifically and in detail. Where did the negative thinking come from? How long have you held on to that notion? How long have you been making that excuse?

Once you've identified all the buts and limiting beliefs in your mind, bring them down to the end of your mental driveway and release them all. Envision a huge garbage truck taking each of those nonserving, outdated, fear-minded buts away for good.

Practice this exercise whenever you need to lighten your load a little. Think of it as your going out of unfinished business sale!

Negative beliefs about yourself and your ability to succeed act as anesthesia to your sense of passion and confidence. They will sabotage your weight-loss efforts if you let them. It is important to work toward getting rid of as many negative thoughts in your mind as you possibly can. Here's an exercise to help you do just that.

In much the same way we use dental floss to clean our teeth, we can use a similar method to clean out our minds. Employing mental floss is a method for removing what is challenging us mentally and emotionally. To do it, you must first identify key habitual thought patterns that continually get in the way of your success. Watch your thoughts, day by day, and start to notice when negative things occur. Then, when those thoughts arise, I want you to remove them from your mind by transferring them to paper. By writing them down, you are better able to see and to disengage them—stare them straight in the eye.

At first it's tricky to even notice they're there, but after a while you'll be on a no-holds-barred thought rampage, and as you key into your mind more and more, you'll also notice that most of these mental messages are reflexive—they seem to come up at the oddest times, for no reason at all. But there is a reason somewhere, and know this, too: even if they seem errant, they will continue to come up and bring you down until you physically remove them and throw them away.

That's why you need to work at flossing your mind throughout your entire day, and as you do, you'll begin to see that your dialogue becomes empowering to you and to those around you, too. It's like becoming electric! You will see that your life quickly begins to reflect more of your true thinking and your true vision for your life. Continue to pay attention to yourself. You can even play games with this exercise to see how long you can go through your day, your week, and your month without being brought down or caught up in a belief or thinking pattern that is no longer true for you. You'll be amazed at what happens. You'll continually be able to go longer and grow stronger with your self-care, and your ability to transcend obstacles will strengthen in new ways.

This has been particularly true of my clients who were especially down or in a place where they had been beating themselves up pretty badly; of those who were very vulnerable to feeding their hurt with less than healthy foods. When they began to use this practice, not only did they quit beating themselves up but they were able to feed themselves with loving, supportive dialogue rather than food. Their hunger was met.

Remember, *you are not your history.* You are the present moment, and that is the greatest and most freeing thing you can ever know. Herein lies your ability to change and grow! Today you have the choice to make your life the way you'd like it to be. From your weight to your attitude to your relationships and how you interact with the world, you can either allow your history and all of its weight and disappointment to continue to direct your life as it always has or you can decide to show up new, open, and willing to let your potential move through you and express itself as you—no more buts about it!

4. Create a Positive Mindset

Consider what would happen if you would renew your thinking to complement and support who you are today as well as where you want to go in the years ahead. What if you allowed all new, positive thoughts to guide and support you every day—how would that be? What if you nurtured a genuine belief in yourself? How would things change?

I tell my patients that your inner atmosphere creates your outer weather. Think about that for a moment. The things we contemplate on the inside are what become us on the outside. If you are holding thoughts that are critical, judgmental, and fault finding within yourself, then you can expect to get exactly the same from the world around you.

On the flip side, the beautiful and empowering truth is that if you envision thoughts that are open, loving, and accepting, that's what you will attract from the world around you. Your perspective casts either shadows or light. And while simply saying "I will lose weight and look beautiful" won't make the pounds melt away, if you make daily strides to become more positive and undertake a complete positive thinking initiative, you can change your life in ways you never imagined.

> The greatest discovery of my generation is that human beings, by changing the inner attitudes of their minds, can change the outer aspects of their lives.
>
> —William James

It's a fact—each morning, you can influence your day right from the start. Do you wake up thinking "Good morning, God!" or do you wake up thinking "Good God, it's morning"? You can imagine which one of these statements sets the course for a more positive day. By just shifting words, you can creatively change your inner dialogue to transform your outer experience.

One of the great challenges in learning to change your inner dialogue from conspiring to inspiring is finding a way to see your thoughts as nourishment. Those things running through your mind are not just empty thoughts without any effect. What you think and believe profoundly influences your life, and you alone have the power to change your frame of mind. You must listen to your inner coach.

When you're trying to lose weight, you can go through myriad emotions and much self-doubt. All too often the loudest voice within you belongs to your inner critic—the one who's always telling you what you're doing wrong and that you're never going to amount to anything. But what if you tuned in to your inner coach instead? Your coach is the part of you who is your true self; the you who is good, loving, and alive with purpose. Up until now, most of us have trained ourselves to listen to the critic, but now it's your coach's turn to speak.

It's time to create a new inner dialogue, a new conversation with yourself. Doing your daily mental flossing to remove negative thoughts will help this process and will help you begin connecting with your positive side. You need to develop a friendship with your heart. Begin listening to it every day. Take time out during your morning or afternoon to listen to the coach inside of you, and actively disregard that inner critic that's usually so loud.

Positivity Props

Methods and techniques for how to surround yourself with people, objects, and experiences that aid and encourage positive change are key to weight-loss success. This exercise is exciting and enlightening.

Simply make an assessment and write down the areas and places in your life where you tend to spend a lot of time. Notice what is good and less than good about these areas. For instance, if you spend a lot of time in your car, ask yourself if what you listen to while you're in it inspires you and adds positivity to your life? If not, what could you be listening to that would bring forth more inspiration? How about placing pictures, quotes, and whatever else brings you joy in the areas where you spend time, like the kitchen or your office workspace?

Surround yourself with positive mental triggers. If you can see it, you can be it!

It takes time to make this change and bring this nurturing voice out. But the beauty and the power of befriending your inner coach is that its power and positive influence surpass just supporting your weight-loss goals. Just think of all the places you could apply its loving support to your life! By listening to your inner coach instead of your critic, you'll care for yourself well. You'll find appreciation for yourself and for your new way of life. You'll find renewed strength.

I fear you may be thinking that it's going to take all the willpower you can muster to keep the bad thoughts away and create a new way of thinking. But actually willpower has nothing to do with it. Let's delete the word *willpower* from our vocabulary. Let's replace it with *willingness*. As you look toward nourishing both your body and mind with healthy foods and attitudes, you need to understand that you're not fighting something but are instead *creating* it. When you move toward building a positive mindset, it isn't about what you won't do but about what you *will* do.

Are you willing to nourish yourself with healthy foods on a daily basis? Are you willing to make movement and exercise consistent entities in your life? When the entire focus of a program is based solely on a very limited goal such as fighting weight or losing inches, you may feel limited—it's you and the scale and how much willpower you have. Your sense of accomplishment and success rests on a rather arbitrary number and it's usually a setup for losing more faith than pounds.

However, it's different with the NutriSystem Nourish program. You're asked to be willing—willing to try new foods; willing to experiment with movement and exercise; willing to ask a friend to join you on the program. Are you willing to go out to dinner and order low-glycemic, healthy portions while your friends or family members order fattening fried foods? Are you willing to prepare your own version of dinner while the rest of the family eats a pizza? Are you willing to rediscover the real you? It's all about being open to what is possible.

Okay, then . . . if you're *willing,* then we can begin setting some new goals!

5. Set New Goals

As part of the NutriSystem Nourish program for weight loss, I recommend setting *whole goals.* Unlike traditional goals, which are usually all set on the outside, whole goals have both an inner and an outer piece to them. For instance, where most diets are concerned, the focus relies too heavily on an outer result. When the goal is simply to lose pounds, experience has shown me that this does not keep us motivated for the long run.

Many times we will reach our goal, and then what do we do? We tend to get away from the plan. Pounds alone will not keep you motivated. Instead, when you set an inner goal—for example, Increase my self-love and confidence or Be a model for health and vitality for my children and spouse or Have energy to play ball with my kids—it is multidimensional and can offer you inspiration for the rest of your life.

I know that when I mention the idea of goal setting, many people respond with less than enthusiastic remarks like, "Goal setting, I've tried that . . . it doesn't work for me," or "Goals are just too out there for me to focus on." I would like to challenge you on that perspective and ask you to try setting goals once again. Goals give us direction, require us to get a plan, and help clear away the distractions in life. They innately make you a clearer, more confident person.

Through your success on this program, you'll realize something very important: you *do* get to choose what you want to do and be. Life is yours to create. But if you don't have a goal in mind, you will wander aimlessly, as if kicking a ball around instead of playing a game with an end in view.

Life Mapping

If you want your environment to support your dreams, try this exercise.

Set aside a window of time, like a few hours one day, to create a powerful life-building model for yourself. Imagine the life of your desires and create a visual that reflects it. Cut out pictures, affirmations, quotes—anything that inspires you visually or verbally—and place them all together in a collage, hanging it in an area in which you spend time daily.

See it, feel it, become it!

So take the time to set some new inspiring goals. Think of them as dreams with a deadline. And pry yourself away from keeping your aspirations in the all-too-familiar and less-than-inspiring realm of pounds lost or just a target weight. Go for something bigger! Establish a goal for experiencing the life of your dreams and do not hold back.

This may feel very uncomfortable at first, and you may feel a bit ridiculous or even foolish for thinking about this kind of goal, but just take a deep breath and stretch into it by envisioning it, writing it down, and seeing it in your mind's eye.

You're worthy of whatever goal you can imagine setting—that's precisely why you can imagine it. So if you ever think, Who am I to set such a goal? let me tell you this: you are most deserving of that goal; you are a living miracle, and within you lies the love, grace, and beauty to go for and realize your highest expression.

Whatever your mind can conceive and believe, your body can achieve!

Your mind is such a powerful tool. That's why you need to think proactively about what you want to carry along with you in life. Are you up for something lighter? Can you think brighter? If you can, you'll transform your life, and through this new mindset, you'll find weight-loss success. The most important thing to remember is that what has happened to you in the past does not matter now. Isn't that a relief? What truly matters is that you are willing to change and start sowing and cultivating the seeds that will reap a tremendous harvest.

You have the power to create a phenomenal life. This is your opportunity, your freedom, and your right. It all starts in your head—mind over matter.

4

Relax Your Mind, Shrink Your Behind!

The Stress/Fat Connection

Too many people live their lives focused on either the past or the future. Are you one of them? If so, you have a great opportunity to use the NutriSystem Nourish program not only to lose weight and feel great but to find peace in "presentness."

With my patients and throughout my own life, I've come to realize that focusing mainly on either the past or the future generally produces unnecessary amounts of anxiety. You're either so busy feeling bad about your past that you can't get past it, or you're too worried about the future to even arrive. Neither is a good situation, especially if you're trying to lose weight.

Together, we just spent the last three chapters discussing how to manage our food intake, our metabolism, and our mindset. These three elements are key to a well-rounded, well-nourished lifestyle and weight-loss effort. But in order to reach your full potential and weight-loss goal, to be successful in all the areas we've talked about so far, you need to do something first—focus on the present and control your stress.

While it's beneficial to learn from the past as well as to be prepared for the future, if you want to reach your potential, life should be lived here in the present, and through focus and true concentration you can do that. It's only once you *are* directly focused on the here and now that you can then ask yourself if you actually want to stay there or move in another direction. Then you can define what stands in the way of your getting there.

I don't mean for you to outline a whole laundry list of all the things that aren't great in your life—like you may not have the fantastic dream job you've always wanted, or your kids or your neighbors sometimes drive you nuts. I'm certainly not suggesting that you up and quit your job, leave your family, or move to another zip code in a quest for ultimate peace and prosperity. You wouldn't find it that way, anyway. Dissatisfaction is usually more about internal factors than external ones, so even if you don't love your job or your house or your schedule or your weight, that in and of itself may have little to do with your actual reason for unhappiness—it's just a symptom of it.

What I *am* saying is that if you're feeling an uneasiness, either a general malaise or an uncontrollable chaoticness about things, *that's* what you need to address. You need to tackle the deeper reasons for what's not working in your life and try to resolve them, or you won't ever be satisfied by any job, household, or person in your life—including yourself. By focusing on the present, you can deal with what's going on with your life, then you'll be poised for success in your weight-loss program because you will be able to truly focus on your food program, eating behaviors, and exercise.

You may be thinking that this is easier said than done. Your life is filled with so much daily stress that you can hardly get through the day, let alone address all of these issues. You are not alone. As a society, we've given in to the notion that unhealthy levels of stress are an undeniable part of the human experience, an incontestable component of living life. I don't accept that, and you shouldn't, either. That's why I've devoted this chapter to stress and how to deal with it. Managing stress is such an important topic and central cornerstone of the NutriSystem Nourish program that I want to spend some time exploring it. Throughout this chapter, I'm going to do two things: explain to you exactly what stress does to your body and how it hinders weight loss and give you concrete solutions for managing it.

We're going to address stress and set it free!

A Day in the Life of NutriSystem Nourish

Theresa follows a combination of the Prepared Foods Meal Plan with the Do-It-Yourself Meal Plan for her weight-loss program.

Theresa is a stay-at-home mom, raising two small children and trying to get back down to her pre-pregnancy weight. It's Friday, and Theresa's 11-month-old serves as her alarm clock bright and early. Within the hour, her household has a happy hum. After getting her husband out the door, she prepares some scrambled egg whites with salsa and splits an orange with her 3-year-old daughter. By 10 A.M., she's got her kids loaded into the van, and is headed to the health club. After settling her little ones in the child care room there, she enjoys a 1-hour yoga and relaxation class—something she's been doing for about 3 months now. Recentered, Theresa stops by the grocery store on the way home to pick up a few items.

While making lunch (a NutriSystem Vegetarian Pasta Salad over fresh spinach leaves and a glass of milk for her; sandwiches for her kids), Theresa chops up the veggies she bought at the store for use tonight and tomorrow in salads. By 1:30 P.M., both kids are napping and Theresa takes 15 minutes to email a friend.

Around 3 P.M., she's outside gardening while her kids play on the lawn, and she snacks on some fresh pear slices and light yogurt. Around 6 P.M., her husband arrives home and they sit down to a great dinner of Thai Chicken with Broccoli (from the NutriSystem Nourish recipes) and some fresh zucchini from their garden. After bathing the kids, everyone gets some Peach Frozen Yogurt (another NutriSystem Nourish recipe), and after many loads of laundry, bedtime follows.

It's been another great day on the NutriSystem Nourish program for Theresa.

Stress Really Is Fattening

Stress can make you fat, and leading a stressful lifestyle can kill your weight-loss efforts. Numerous studies have concluded that chronic stress definitely leads to overeating because it has a direct relationship to appetite. See if you can relate to this scenario: You sit down to pay your bills one night and realize the budget is a bit tighter than you thought. You wake up the next morning, and while still stressed out about your money situation, you dash out the door, knowing you'll be late for work because you have a sick child and you have just been notified that your meeting has been moved up a half-hour. While you're rushing around, you're probably not even thinking of eating. After you take your son to the doctor, drop him off at your mother's house, and get the meeting behind you—basically get all the acute stress down to a low roar—*now* you want to eat, and boy, you're not craving broccoli!

When you're stressed, you usually eat more food, and more poorly, too. But did you know that your body chemistry has everything to do with that?

During the initial phase of stress, certain hormones are released to suppress appetite, but then later in the stress response another hormone is released to reencourage that appetite—to boost it back up again. This secondary hormone is *cortisol*, and it's an important one to know about.

The Cortisol Connection

Released from the adrenal gland, cortisol gives your body the ability to run, fight, and expend energy—the fight-or-flight mechanism. The problem is that in today's hectic world we rarely do this; we rarely actually fight and make flight or expend enough of the energy that's produced. Instead, we tend to sit with our stress either in our cars while caught in traffic, in front of our computers, or while watching TV, wishing the world would go away. We stress, we sit, and we eat, in that order. And because we're not expending that energy after stressful events, cortisol levels remain high for hours in our system, which in turn means that we have an appetite fueled by cortisol for hours, too. And that's not a good thing.

Enter cortisol's sibling, insulin. When cortisol levels rise, insulin levels also rise, and, as you now know, they work to do their main job, which is maintaining blood sugar levels in the body. But insulin also enables sugar storage in the liver and muscle cells and fat storage in the fat cells. That's how stress makes you fat. When you are chronically stressed, you burn fewer calories, you lose muscle, and you experience an increase in appetite, and it's usually for highly refined, high-glycemic, sugary carbohydrates. You eat them, and your body in turn stores their sugars as fat.

When excessive stress causes cortisol levels to rise, that in turn causes other hormone levels to drop. Because of these hormonal fluctuations, many other normal body functions may be inhibited. Increased cortisol levels can also lead to loss of muscle, and loss of muscle decreases metabolism, increases your risk for diseases, and accelerates aging.

Additionally, when you experience stress, there is a real physical and chemical demand placed on your brain's ability to balance other hormones and neurotransmitters (chemicals that transmit nerve impulses in the brain). Any deficiency of these brain chemical messengers can result in a variety of potentially debilitating symptoms.

Another result of your brain's inability to balance neurotransmitters can be lower levels of another hormone, dopamine. Lack of dopamine can lead to a sluggish metabolism, impaired concentration, and lack of motivation.

Still other neurotransmitters are helpful in creating a sense of balance, peace, and mental harmony.

Cortisol also appears to interfere with the ability of the body to absorb calcium, which can lead to weight gain and osteoporosis. It suppresses energy, exhausts the adrenal system, and leads to an increased susceptibility to disease.

In a nutshell, having a high cortisol level is not good for your body.

How can you lower your cortisol levels? From a purely physical perspective, to control cortisol levels in your bloodstream you need to balance your diet and watch those foods you fuel your body with. The NutriSystem Nourish program is a perfect way to begin balancing your diet and warding off high cortisol levels in your bloodstream. Because this program integrates the necessary dietary factors needed to help lower cortisol—like eating low-glycemic foods, proper portion sizes and frequent meals—with lifestyle practices to help you manage stress better and an exercise and movement plan, you get a complete, well-rounded, and proven approach to solving the problem of stress.

The program is so easy to follow (the NutriSystem Nourish prepared foods cook in minutes and fit into your daily routine) that this alone can eliminate a significant amount of stress in your life. In a published university study on dieting with prepared foods, scientists found that prepared, portion-controlled foods do, in fact, help people lose weight more effectively. By following the NutriSystem Nourish program and by cooking the easy-to-prepare foods yourself and/or utilizing the new NutriSystem Nourish ready-to-go prepared foods, you will be effectively supporting a healthy response to stress and normalizing your levels of cortisol.

Blow Stress Off

When we look to begin controlling stress in our lives, we need first to give our bodies the best possible foundation for dealing with it. Breathing, meditation, and yoga are three excellent building blocks for this foundation. Let's talk about breathing first.

A key solution lies in monitoring your breathing. That sounds simple enough, right? Sometimes it's a little easier said than done. You will notice that when you are feeling stressed or frightened, you tend to take shallow breaths. This simple act can create a landslide of undesirable effects, including an increase in the stress hormones being released in your body, which can drive many diet derailing scenarios, including cravings for sugar, anxiety, and even depression. In contrast, when you breathe properly from your belly and diaphragm, you promote life-affirming chemistry that is energizing and confidence building. And here's the best news: you can practice healthy breathing all day, every day, and enjoy its powerful results for the rest of your life!

Shallow breathing, which the majority of people do these days, produces the release of stress hormones and cortisol. When under stress, as so many of us are, it seems natural to take shorter, shallower breaths, but it is actually the worst thing you can possibly do. Inefficient breathing initiates the stress response. The control boards for both respiration and the fight-or-flight response are located in the limbic system of the brain. Our bodies interpret short breaths as a first-level response to danger. Anytime we move to shallow breathing, we create a catalyst for our system to think we're under stress.

The most effective solution to shallow breathing that I've found does not come in the form of a pill, a therapist, a massage, or any other relaxing luxury. It comes from simply using your lungs to their fullest capacity. Breathe deeply. Doing so reverses the damage done by breathing feebly: it lowers blood lactate levels, puts a halt to excessive production of cortisol, encourages a healthier potassium/sodium balance and an alkaline environment in the body, and lowers your blood pressure. In essence, it does a body good!

Every breath is another opportunity to relieve stress and lower cortisol levels so that your body can lose more weight. Use your belly. When you take a deep breath and bring it down into your diaphragm, it causes your mind and body to say, "Ahhh, good . . . everything's okay." Less stress, more fat burning.

Breathing Techniques

We have literally forgotten how to breathe—and not just under pressure but all the time. Many of us neglect to breathe well, day after day. When we do remember to inhale and exhale well, instead of doing so slowly and in a relaxed manner—using the whole torso to take in oxygen and letting the belly rise and fall with each breath like bellows, or a sleeping baby or animal—we confine respiration to our collarbone area. This cheats the body of one of its most essential functions.

Poor posture, lack of mindfulness, and stress are the greatest culprits

Breath Work and Abdominal Techniques for Beginners

Your breath is your key to life. Your abdominals—the muscles that support proper breathing—span the area between the breastbone (sternum) and the pubic bone. By performing these breathing exercises you will learn to locate and tone theses muscles, ultimately enhancing the resting tone of your abdominal muscles.

Begin breathing exercises either sitting forward on the edge of a chair or lying flat on your back with a small bolster or rolled-up towel under your knees for support. Lengthen your spine so that your back is not resting against the back of the chair but rather is perpendicular to the floor. Your feet should be about hip width apart. Sit up tall and look straight ahead. If you are lying down, you can still maintain the sensation of lengthening your spine and gaze upward straight above your nose.

Begin to notice your breath. Notice that your abdominal wall expands when you inhale. Your abdominal wall softens or falls when you exhale. Place both hands on your belly below your navel. Your fingers should be pointing towards your pubic bone. Inhale and allow your belly to expand into your hands. As you exhale, gently use your hands to pull your abdominal muscles up and in, sort of like zipping up a pair of pants. Repeat this 5 times, then rest and relax the abdominal muscles and maintain the length of the spine. Start again, and this time do a set of 4, then rest. Repeat this exercise often.

contributing to shallow breathing. Rounding the shoulders and letting the chest cave in, which happens when you don't sit or stand with an elongated spine, crushes the lungs and doesn't allow them to expand for each breath, and it doesn't allow room in the abdominal cavity for the diaphragm to drop, making more room for the lungs. When we are nervous or anxious, we go into a posture of self-defense, clenching the stomach and chest muscles. We hold tension in the back and shoulders and this constricts lung capacity.

Here's one way to develop good breathing habits: Take 5 minutes every hour to breathe deeply—*really* deeply. Stop whatever you're doing at some point each hour and breathe five full breaths in a row. This is great for productivity. A breathing practice lowers cortisol and helps the brain to initiate a wonderfully relaxed but not sedate state that allows for focus and concentration. If you work on your breathing before an important meeting, you will be present, more focused, and more alert. In terms of everyday life, by fortifying your mind with adequate oxygen, you will enjoy a sharper ability to make the right decisions about things that affect your health and happiness—like whether you should have that giant candy bar or a healthier chicken breast for lunch.

Here's another breathing technique you can try: Breathe in deeply through your nose, hold, and count to 10, then exhale slowly through your mouth. Do this several times. It's one of the oldest tricks in the book, but it is one of the most underused and underrated stress-relieving tactics around.

The key to allowing your body to breathe deeply is not just to focus on the breath and correct your posture but also to allow the body to soften, to be in a more open and receptive mode to what's being taken in. Focusing or meditating on your breath can create this receptiveness, and by doing breathing exercises you will also remain focused on the present, minimizing anger about the past or anxiety about the future.

Other techniques that aid in creating presentness include meditation and yoga.

Give Yourself a Time-Out

Meditation takes the brain out of a restless state by simply letting it rest. It gives the brain an opportunity to step back and replenish itself, which is key, because an overextended mind is a stressed-out mind. We are a culture of overdoers who take pride in being able to keep several balls in the air at once. We simultaneously do business, eat, and drive; we watch the news while we study; we read or talk on the phone while we exercise or listen to the radio; and we eat breakfast while we're getting ready for work. It's simply crazy. Trying to do too many things at once can lead to a very scattered sense of being, to feelings of being overwhelmed and disconnected, and ultimately to stress. And stress makes you fat.

When we step out of that active *doing* mode by practicing various modes of meditation, the brain picks up the clues that it doesn't have to perform. It takes time to recalibrate, regroup, and replenish itself.

Yoga and meditation are critically important means to this end. They're both built on the idea of mindfulness and the ability to focus the mind on the breath, a thought, or an affirmation. Both enhance the mind–body connection and keep the mind from wandering. Practicing mindfulness and

Meditation 101

Meditation doesn't need to be some long, drawn-out, time-consuming practice. You can choose to meditate almost anywhere for any amount of time. For example, you can meditating by simply being aware of your breathing. A relaxed full breath form your belly is the beginning of the journey to lowered stress and cortisol levels and increased peace.

To incorporate meditation and relaxation into your day, I suggest trying a morning practice of meditation centered around trust and faith, breathing in while focusing on these things and releasing doubt and worry. In the evenings you can meditate on gratitude and acceptance. Each time, simply sit in a comfortable position, or if you prefer, lie down on your back, allowing your body to fully surrender to relaxation, releasing all busy thinking. Let go of any self-defeating thoughts and open to your true self—the self that is perfect, whole, and at peace. Allow each breath to move fully down into your belly, filling it slowly and completely. Repeat these deep breaths for as long as you like; 10 to 15 minutes is a good starting practice.

bringing awareness to the breath are the most effective ways to regain balance psychologically, physiologically, and spiritually.

When I talk about meditation or yoga practice, it has nothing to do with being in a trance or becoming involved with any religious sect. Meditation is basically the same thing as focused contemplation, introspection, or taking a quiet moment. Meditation or mindfulness is about being present, focused, and centered. It's about disciplining the mind, enhancing mental clarity, and boosting energy.

One of the greatest gifts from yoga or meditative practices is that you can create mental and emotional space. If you nurture that space and maintain it, no one—no amount of work or stress—can take that away from you. Plus, when you meditate on an emotion or a quality such as joy or gratitude, it in turn enlarges your capacity and facility to experience and recognize that feeling. It's utterly amazing.

Meditation can prime you spiritually for optimism and possibility. It also works on your body chemistry to make happiness and balance more accessible for you physiologically. In combination with attention to the breath, meditation lowers the production of stress hormones in the body, encourages an alkaline environment that discourages disease, and lowers blood lactate, which is associated with anxiety. And all that from just slowing down, focusing, and breathing.

Go Yoga

To increase energy, balance, flexibility, and overall health, no form of exercise is more effective than yoga. For some, the very thought of yoga brings up images of bodies bent into pretzels and other uncomfortable positions. Or the word *yoga* itself may bring along connotations of New Age–ism or a far-out mentality. All of these are off base, since the practice of yoga is simply meditation at its active, moving best, and it's gaining huge recognition by professional athletes, businesspeople, expectant moms, and regular people all over. People are simply starting to wake up to and recognize all of the health benefits that a consistent practice of yoga can offer—and they're very far-reaching.

I have both personally and professionally witnessed health breakthroughs all brought about through yoga practice.

> When Dr. James first suggested yoga to me as part of my weight-loss program, I immediately pictured skinny people who were blessed with bodies that could do very unnatural things. At first, it did feel awkward, but I stayed with it. I noticed that I was losing weight, but more so, I noticed that I began to lose something much heavier. I had spent much of my life carrying around the pain of unrelenting self-judgment. My yoga practice has given me the peace and flexibility to accept myself as I am now—a thinner, happier me.
> —Sherri, age 35

Yoga is very effective in reducing stress, building endurance and strength, improving posture, strengthening the spine, and improving circulation and respiratory function. It can improve the healthy functioning of all body systems including digestion and the cardiovascular system. Yoga works wonders!

Heathful Yoga Hints

- Do yoga in a quiet setting.
- Try yoga at the beginning of the day before you get busy.
- Wear loose-fitting clothing.
- Stretch your muscles. When done correctly, yoga movements should not be painful.
- Quiet your mind so that it can focus.

The many health benefits of yoga are truly powerful, but often the less physical benefits are even more profound, as the practice of yoga can build and strengthen your spirit. A consistent, committed practice of yoga can be an empowering elixir to self-esteem. Exploring intentional movement and holding positions can develop awareness and help us move through both physical and mental blocks.

Like any exercise program and as when you're developing any skill, yoga is a practice that needs to be learned. I've included a whole routine of easy-to-do yoga in Chapter Seven, and there are also some excellent yoga home videos on the market today. Many health clubs and studios offer a variety of yoga classes (both individual and group) to meet a wide variety of needs.

I recommend giving yourself at least two sessions per week, 20 minutes each, to experience the many gifts that yoga can bring to you and your life. When you think about it, that's less than 1 hour a week spent on an activity that will nourish your entire body and soul—that's quite a bargain!

Creating Bookends

Often, the only time we have to truly be in charge of our daily lives is early in the morning and right before bedtime. These are times when we can create our own rituals.

Starting today, begin to give yourself an extra 10 to 15 minutes in the morning and 10 to 15 minutes in the evening. These are your daily "bookends."

Start your bookend exercise before you even get out of bed by performing 20 deep-belly breaths each morning. Allow yourself to come into the day gently with soft light, gentle music, soothing herbal tea, or a good book. Then take an invigorating walk. At night, do something similar for 15 minutes prior to going to bed, except for the invigorating walk. Dim the lights or light some candles, as this prepares your body chemistry for a sleeping state. (Be sure to blow the candles out when you're ready to sleep.)

Think of your bookends as a hug—one arm in the morning and another arm in the evening—wrapping around your successes of the day and supporting you where you are.

See Chapter 7 for a complete bookend routine.

Whether it's yoga or simple meditation, you'll find that when you practice them consistently, the relaxation response comes more and more quickly. Create a setting around your practice to ritualize it. For example, light a scented candle and play some soothing music every time you start meditating or practicing yoga. This is important because eventually these props will set off a Pavlov-like response in your brain. Your body will know that relaxation is to follow and will begin to settle in before you even start.

There are many different ways to meditate. Whether you begin practicing yoga or simply initiate some of the basic meditation techniques I've offered in this book, you'll be doing yourself a world of good. Just start by finding a time, place, and style that's right for you. For starters, the best way to incorporate meditation and mindfulness into your day-to-day routine may be to schedule it into your bookends, developing a morning and evening practice. On top of that, I'd recommend doing some of the more succinct mindfulness exercises throughout your day. But no matter what approach appeals to you, try it at least for a week or two. I promise that it will truly put you in a completely different state of mind in as little as a few days. See for yourself!

Seeking Courage in the Battle of the Bulge?

Become a warrior!

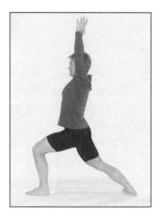

The *warrior pose* is a yoga posture for supporting courage and conviction. Try it the next time you find yourself in a tough spot like the cookie aisle, in front of the dessert cart, or in the face of your refrigerator. Simply move into the warrior pose and empower your courage!

An entire yoga routine is shown in Chapter Seven.

Rewards of Relaxation

Learning to relax and destress can create peace and focus in your life. If you can consciously work to discover what gives you joy and give yourself permission to do more of that, you will be much more at peace with everything you do.

Nourishing Minutes

Living a busy life? No time to nourish yourself? Here are some practices that even the busiest among us can do throughout the day to replenish and nurture.

If you have 1 minute:

- Brush your hair.
- Visualize your favorite vacation.
- Give yourself a temple massage.
- Hold hands with someone.

If you have 5 minutes:

- Read inspirational quotes.
- Breathe deeply in through your nose and out through your mouth.
- Enjoy a cold washcloth on your forehead.

If you have 10 minutes:

- Make an entry in your journal.
- Buy yourself flowers.
- Enjoy a sunrise or sunset.

If you have 20 minutes:

- Light a scented candle.
- Paint your nails a new color.
- Read to a child.

If you have 30 minutes:

- Take a bubble bath.
- Write a letter or email to an old friend.
- Have green tea with a neighbor.

There will always be challenges in life. We all have lackluster tasks and obligations. But if you can find focus and centeredness amidst the busy-craziness of everyday life, the innate challenges become much more doable. By incorporating the lifestyle techniques of the NutriSystem Nourish program into your life, you can streamline your objectives, simplify your life, and manage stress better, which translates into more time for yourself and a higher quality of time for yourself and those you love.

Focusing on the positive in life and clearing your mind on a day-to-day basis takes mental and physical discipline, but the rewards are tremendous. Half the battle against mental restlessness, pessimism, and anxiety can be won by reducing errant thoughts and reflexes, and increasing the focus you put on yourself and what you want out of life. And through this, improved weight loss can be achieved.

When you relax your mind, you actually *can* shrink your behind!

PART TWO

Nourishing Meal Plans

5

NutriSystem Nourish
Meal Plans
Step-by-Step Meal Plan Options

This chapter outlines the heart of the new NutriSystem Nourish weight-loss program—the NutriSystem Nourish Meal Plans. This program was specially designed to jumpstart your metabolism by fueling your body frequently with the optimum balance of low-glycemic carbohydrates, proteins, healthy fats, and fiber so that you avoid low blood sugar levels and hunger and keep your body burning fat at peak levels. This plan even helps you monitor your portions.

It's all here and ready to help you lose up to 17 pounds in the first 4 weeks and a safe and healthy 1 to 2½ pounds each week thereafter. Simply choose from one of the two NutriSystem Nourish Meal Plan options—or any combination of the two that works best for you—to get started:

1. *Do-It-Yourself Meal Plan:* This plan features foods you fix for yourself at home or eat out at restaurants and incorporates several of the delicious low-glycemic recipes found in Chapter Nine of this book. Each of these recipes indicates the estimated time it will take to make them so that you can plan according to your individual schedule for the day. There are 28 days of sample menus outlined that you can follow, as well as guidelines for servings and portion sizes.

2. *Prepared Foods Meal Plan:* This plan features the new NutriSystem Nourish prepared foods that you purchase from NutriSystem (log on to nutrisystem.com or call 1-800-321-THIN), along with fresh grocery fruits and vegetables that you add in. Each day, you simply choose your

breakfast, lunch, and dinner entrees plus a dessert from the many convenient and tasty NutriSystem Nourish foods that only take minutes to cook. You don't need to think about monitoring your low-glycemic carbohydrates, fats, proteins, calories, or even portions—these things are already done for you with this plan. Just choose your foods and start losing weight!

You may follow either one of these plans entirely—doing everything yourself or using the NutriSystem Nourish foods exclusively—or you can combine the two plans. Some people use the Prepared Foods Meal Plan during the week and incorporate the Do-It-Yourself Meal Plan and low-glycemic recipes on the weekends when they have more time. Others find it easier to make their own breakfasts and lunches but enjoy a NutriSystem Nourish prepared entree for dinner. It all works. This program was designed to be flexible enough to meet your individual needs. You simply choose or design a meal plan that fits your individual lifestyle and eating occasions.

Daily Meal Plan Overview

Before we dive into the two meal plans, here's an overview of how both of them work. On both plans, your daily meals will include:

- Low-fat protein at each meal
- 3 or more servings of cooked or raw vegetables
- 2 or 3 fruit servings
- 2 or 3 high-calcium dairy foods
- 2 to 4 low-glycemic whole-grain or bean servings (or more, depending on your caloric needs)
- 1 to 2 servings of heart-healthy fats added to your vegetables or salads or used in cooking. Look for monounsaturated or polyunsaturated oils such as canola oil, olive oil, safflower oil, peanut oil, or sunflower oil. Other heart-healthy fats are found in avocado, nuts and olives. Typical serving sizes are 1 teaspoon oil, 1 teaspoon mayonnaise, 2 tablespoons low-fat salad dressing, or 1 tablespoon nuts. Avoid margarine, shortening, and other hardened fats that include trans fats in the form of partially hydrogenated vegetable oils.

You must nourish your body each day with five eating times—three meals plus two snacks. Distributing your foods evenly throughout the day maintains normal blood sugar and energy levels. This will help you increase your metabolism, control your appetite, and lose weight.

The number of servings and calories appropriate for your individual weight loss can vary based on weight, gender, and activity level. Generally, men need more calories than women, so we've divided our plans accordingly. However, if you are significantly overweight or very active, you may need more servings than are listed in the sample menus. For help choosing a plan or if you have any questions, you can call 1-800-321-THIN or email NutriSystem at info@nutrisystem.com to speak with a professional counselor. There is never any cost—no membership or sign-up fees—for any NutriSystem support service.

Regardless of which meal plan you choose, here's a look at what your daily plan and eating schedule will be. It shows you the breakdown of how many servings of each individual food group you should have to keep your metabolism burning at its optimal level.

NutriSystem Nourish Daily Meal Plan Overview

	Protein	Dairy	Fruit	Vegetable	Grains	Fat
Breakfast	(● or ●)		●		●	
Lunch	●			●	●	●
Snack		●	●			
Dinner	●			●●	●	●
Snack		●	(● or ●)			

● = 1 serving

Wherever you see a dot, you eat a serving of that food group. You may wonder how much is a serving. Leave it to NutriSystem to help with that.

Perfect Portions™

For decades, NutriSystem has been helping people learn the right portion sizes. Here are the recommended serving sizes for each food group.

Vegetables

Include several servings of vegetables daily for the phytonutrients and fiber benefits. Unless noted serving size is ½ cup cooked or 1 cup raw.

Artichoke (½)

Asparagus

Bean sprouts

Bok choy

Broccoli

Brussels sprouts

Cabbage

Carrots

Cauliflower

Collard Greens

Eggplant

Green beans

Jicama, raw (½ cup)

Kale

Kohlrabi

Leeks

Mushrooms

Mustard greens

Okra

Onions

Pea pods

Peppers

Rutabaga

Spaghetti squash

Spinach

Summer squash

Tomato (1 medium)

Turnip greens

Turnips

Water chestnuts

Zucchini

Salad Vegetables

One or two of your vegetable servings can be unlimited amounts of raw salad vegetables including leafy greens such as lettuce, romaine, spinach, endive, cucumbers, zucchini, celery, mushrooms, radishes, or cabbage.

Fruits

Whole fruits are vastly preferable to juices since they provide more fiber.

Apple (1 small)

Applesauce (½ cup)

Apricots (4 halves or ½ cup)

Banana (½ of 9")

Blackberries (¾ cup)

Blueberries (¾ cup)

Cantaloupe (1 cup cubes or ⅓ melon)

Cherries (12)

Cranberries, dried (2 Tbsp.)

Figs (2)

Grapefruit (½)

Grapes (15)

Honeydew melon (⅛ medium or 1 cup cubes)

Kiwi (1 large)

Mandarin oranges (½ cup)

Mango (½ medium)

Nectarine (1 medium)

Orange (1 medium)

Peach (½ cup or 2 halves)

Pear (1 small)

Pineapple, canned (⅓ cup)

Pineapple, fresh (¾ cup)

Plums (2)

Prunes (3)

Raisins (2 Tbsp.)

Raspberries (1cup)

Strawberries (1¼ cups)

Tangerines (2)

Grains/Beans/Bread

Whole-grain bread products and beans have lower glycemic index values than more refined grain products.

Bagel, whole-grain or rye (½ small)

Barley (1/3 cup)

Beans, garbanzo, pinto, kidney, white, split or black-eyed peas (⅓ cup)

Bread, whole-wheat, oatmeal, pumpernickel, rye, sourdough (1 slice)

Buckwheat groats (½ cup)

Bulgur (½ cup)

Cereal, All-Bran (½ cup)

Cereals, high fiber and high protein such as granola, muesli (¼ to ⅓ cup)

Cookies, low-fat, low-sugar such as oatmeal or whole-wheat (1 small)

Corn (½ cup)

Couscous (⅓ cup)

Crackers, whole-grain or rye (¾ oz.)

English muffin, whole-wheat (½)

Melba toast, rye or pumpernickel (5 oblong)

Oatmeal, rolled or steel cut (½ cup)

Pasta, cooked al dente (½ cup)

Pita, whole-grain (½ of 6")

Potato, new or red-skinned (½ cup)

Rice, basmati (⅓ cup)

Rice, brown (⅓ cup)

Roll, whole-grain (1 small)

Rye wafers (3)

Rye Krisp (3 triple crackers)

Sweet potato (⅓ cup)

Quinoa (⅓ cup)

Wild rice (½ cup)

Yam (⅓ cup)

Fat Servings

Select from these heart-healthy fats.

Avocado (⅛)

Mayonnaise (1 tsp.)

Mayonnaise, light (2 tsp.)

Nuts

Almonds (6)

Cashews (5)

Nuts *(continued)*

Peanuts (10 large)

Pecans (5 halves)

Pine nuts (1 Tbsp)

Pistachios (15)

Walnuts (4 halves)

Peanut butter (1 tsp.)

Oil, canola, olive, peanut, corn, safflower (1 tsp.)

Olives (5 large)

Salad dressings, regular (1 Tbsp.)

Salad dressings, reduced-fat (2 Tbsp.)

Seeds, sesame, pumpkin, sunflower (1Tbsp)

Tahini (1 tsp.)

Milk/Dairy Servings

Dairy servings provide calcium necessary for healthy bones and teeth. Calcium also helps promote weight loss and lower blood pressure.

Fat-free or 1% milk (8 oz.)

Light or fat-free Yogurt (8 oz.)

Low-fat soy milk (calcium-fortified) (8 oz.)

Lactaid milk (8 oz.)

Buttermilk (8 oz.)

Fat-free or low-fat Cheese (1 oz.)

Nonfat or low-fat cottage cheese (¼ cup)

Parmesan, grated (2 Tbsp.)

Ricotta cheese, low-fat (¼ cup)

Protein Servings

Adequate but not excessive protein at each meal is important to controlling appetite and meeting the body's needs for essential amino acids.

Limit dinner portions to approximately 4 to 6 ounces (palm size) of low-fat protein foods. Recommended lunch portions are approximately 2 to 4 ounces.

Breakfast protein can include 1 egg or 3 egg whites or 1 ounce lean meat or smoked fish or whey or soy shakes.

Meats, poultry, and seafood should be baked, broiled, steamed, not fried.

Chicken or turkey, skinless

Lean beef—flank steak, tenderloin, round

Fish, fresh, frozen, or smoked, such as lox or tuna canned in water

Shellfish, shrimp, scallops, clams, lobster, crabmeat

Tofu, tempeh

Soy protein vegetarian foods, veggie burger, sausage or veggie dogs

Eggs, egg whites, and egg substitutes

Lean pork—tenderloin, boiled or baked ham, lean pork chop

Game meats, venison, buffalo

Lamb, lean shoulder, cubes, sirloin

Veal, chop or roast

Whey or soy powder

NutriSystem Nourish Meal Plans

NutriSystem Nourish Do-It-Yourself Meal Plan

This plan uses all homemade and fresh foods and works best for those who enjoy cooking their own foods.

For ease in menu planning, we have included 28 days worth of sample menus made from NutriSystem Nourish recipes and common restaurant or home-cooked foods. The dishes within each day can certainly be rearranged to fit your schedule and appetite. For instance, you can switch the lunch and dinner meals around or replace the fruit suggestions with your favorites. You also do not need to follow the outlined days in any particular order. Variation is the key so that your taste buds will always be intrigued.

Do-It-Yourself Meal Plan I—Sample Menus

Day 1	Women's Plan	Men's Plan
Breakfast:		
All-Bran Cereal	½ cup	1 cup
Fresh Strawberries	1¼ cups	1¼ cups
Fat-free Milk	1 cup	1 cup
Lunch:		
Turkey	2 oz.	3 oz.
Marinated Cucumbers in fat-free dressing	unlimited	unlimited
Whole-Wheat Bread	1 slice	2 slices
Snack:		
Pear	1 small	1 small
String Cheese	1 oz.	1 oz.
Dinner:		
Sautéed Sea Scallops	4 oz.	6 oz.
Bulgur and Mushroom Pilaf	⅓ cup	⅔ cup
Snow Peas	1 cup	1 cup

Snack:

Prunes	3	3
Light Yogurt	1 cup	1 cup

Day 2	Women's Plan	Men's Plan
Breakfast:		
Steel-cut Oat Porridge	½ cup	1 cup
Dried Cranberries	2 Tbsp.	2 Tbsp.
Fat-free Milk	1 cup	1 cup
Lunch:		
Lean Corned Beef Round	2 oz.	3 oz.
Rye Bread	1 slice	2 slices
Baby Carrots	1 cup	1 cup
Snack:		
Grapes	15	15
Low-fat Cheese	1 oz.	1 oz.
Dinner:		
Grilled Shrimp	4 oz.	6 oz.
Herbed Couscous	⅓ cup	⅔ cup
Stir-Fried Zucchini and Yellow Squash	1 cup	1 cup
Snack:		
Fresh Strawberries	1¼ cups	1¼ cups
Low-fat Ricotta Cheese	¼ cup	¼ cup

Day 3	Women's Plan	Men's Plan
Breakfast:		
Omelet	1 egg + 2 whites	1 egg + 3 whites
Spinach and Mushrooms	¼ cup	¼ cup
Sourdough Toast	1 slice	2 slices
Lunch:		
Grilled Chicken	2 oz.	3 oz.
Cherry Tomatoes	6	6
Romaine Lettuce with 2 T Low-fat Dressing	unlimited	unlimited
Whole-Wheat Crackers	¾ oz.	1½ oz.
Snack:		
Blueberries	¾ cup	¾ cup
Cottage Cheese	¼ cup	¼ cup

Dinner:

Broiled Salmon	4 oz.	6 oz.
Curried Basmati Rice	⅓ cup	⅔ cup
Baked Eggplant	1 cup	1 cup

Snack:

Apricots, fresh or canned in juice	½ cup	½ cup
Light Vanilla Yogurt	1 cup	1 cup

Day 4	Women's Plan	Men's Plan

Breakfast:

Smoked Salmon	1 oz.	2 oz.
Honeydew Cubes	1 cup	1 cup
Whole-grain Bagel	½	1

Lunch:

Crustless Quiche Lorraine (see recipe)	1 serving	1 serving
Mesclun Salad with 2 T Low-fat Dressing	unlimited	unlimited
Pumpernickel Roll	1 small	2 small

Snack:

Apple	1 small	1 small
Fat-free Milk	1 cup	1 cup

Dinner:

Broiled Flank Steak	4 oz.	6 oz.
New Red-skin Potatoes	½ cup	1 cup
Baked Spaghetti Squash	1 cup	1 cup

Snack:

Mini Strawberry Sundae (see recipe)	1 serving	1 serving

Day 5	Women's Plan	Men's Plan

Breakfast:

Low-fat Granola	⅓ cup	⅔ cup
Fresh Raspberries	1 cup	1 cup
Light Vanilla Yogurt	1 cup	1 cup

Lunch:

Tuna Salad made with light mayonnaise	½ cup	¾ cup
Tomato	medium	medium
Romaine Lettuce	unlimited	unlimited
Rye Krisps	1 triple cracker	2 triple crackers

Snack:

Red Grapes	15	15
Fat-free Milk	1 cup	1 cup

Dinner:

Baked Chicken Breast	4 oz.	6 oz.
Herbed Wild Rice	½ cup	1 cup
Green Beans	1 cup	1 cup

Snack:

Flan (see recipe)	1 serving	1 serving

Day 6	Women's Plan	Men's Plan

Breakfast:

Chocolate Banana Smoothie (see recipe)	1 serving	1 serving

Lunch:

Low-fat Veggie Hot Dog	1	2
Carrot and Celery Sticks	unlimited	unlimited
Whole-Grain Roll	1	2

Snack:

Fresh Pineapple Chunks	¾ cup	¾ cup
Cottage Cheese	¼ cup	¼ cup

Dinner:

Baked Flounder	4 oz.	6 oz.
Pasta Shells al dente	½ cup	1 cup
Steamed Spinach	1 cup	1 cup

Snack:

Basmati Rice Pudding (see recipe)	1 serving	1 serving

Day 7	Women's Plan	Men's Plan

Breakfast:

Low-fat Swiss Cheese	1 oz.	2 oz.
Tomato	1 medium	1 medium
Whole-grain English Muffin	½	1

Lunch:

Imitation Crab Salad with light mayonnaise	4 oz.	6 oz.
Mixed Green Salad with 2 T Low-fat Dressing	unlimited	unlimited
Whole-Wheat Bread	1 slice	2 slices

Snack:

Apple	1 small	1 small
Fat-free Milk	1 cup	1 cup

Dinner:

Roasted Pork Tenderloin	4 oz.	6 oz.
Sweet Potato or Yam	⅓ cup	⅔ cup
Mustard Greens	1 cup	1 cup

Snack:

Peanut Butter Cookie (see recipe)	1	1

Day 8	Women's Plan	Men's Plan

Breakfast:

High-Protein, High-Fiber Cereal	¾ cup	1½ cups
Banana, 9"	½	½
Fat-free Milk	1 cup	1 cup

Lunch:

Veggie Burger	1	1
Romaine Lettuce and Sliced Tomatoes	unlimited	unlimited
Multigrain Roll	1	1

Snack:

Grapes	15	15
Low-fat Swiss Cheese	1 oz.	1 oz.

Dinner:

Stir-Fried Tofu	6 oz.	8 oz.
Brown Rice	⅓ cup	⅔ cup
Asparagus	1 cup	1 cup

Snack:

Peach Frozen Yogurt (see recipe)	1 serving	1 serving

Day 9	Women's Plan	Men's Plan

Breakfast:

Mango Lassi (see recipe)	1 serving	1 serving

Lunch:

Chicken Wrap, Black Bean Salsa	1 small	1 medium
Cucumbers and Radishes	unlimited	unlimited

Snack:

Pear	1 small	1 small
Fat-free Yogurt	1 cup	1 cup

Dinner:

Teriyaki Beef and Broccoli (see recipe)	1 serving	1 serving
Brown Rice	$\frac{1}{3}$ cup	$\frac{2}{3}$ cup

Snack:

Oat Bran Pretzels	$\frac{3}{4}$ oz.	$1\frac{1}{2}$ oz.
String Cheese	1 oz.	2 oz.

Day 10	Women's Plan	Men's Plan

Breakfast:

Tropical Piña Smoothie (see recipe)	1 serving	1 serving

Lunch:

Low-fat Greek Salad with Feta and 2 T Low-fat Dressing	small	medium
Whole-Wheat Pita	$\frac{1}{2}$	1

Snack:

Fresh Cherries	12	12
String Cheese	1 oz.	1 oz.

Dinner:

Roast Turkey Breast	4 oz.	6 oz.
Yam	$\frac{1}{3}$ cup	$\frac{2}{3}$ cup
Braised Cabbage	1 cup	1 cup

Snack:

Fresh Figs	2 medium	2 medium
Light Yogurt	1 cup	1 cup

Day 11	Women's Plan	Men's Plan

Breakfast:

Scrambled Egg Whites	3	4
Salsa	2 Tbsp.	2 Tbsp.
Grapefruit	$\frac{1}{2}$	$\frac{1}{2}$
Oatmeal Toast	1 slice	2 slices

Lunch:

Lean Ham Slices	2 oz.	3 oz.
Coleslaw made with light mayo	1 cup	1 cup
Rye Bread	1 slice	2 slices

Snack:

Mango	$\frac{1}{2}$	$\frac{1}{2}$
Light Vanilla Yogurt	1 cup	1 cup

Dinner:

Cheese Ravioli with Tomato Basil Sauce (see recipe)	1 serving	1 serving
Endive Salad with 2 T Low-fat Dressing	unlimited	unlimited

Snack:

Fresh Strawberries	1¼ cups	1¼ cups
Low-fat Ricotta Cheese	¼ cup	¼ cup

Day 12	Women's Plan	Men's Plan

Breakfast:

Poached Egg	1	2
Orange	1	1
Rye Toast	1 slice	2 slices

Lunch:

Savory Lentil Soup (see recipe)	1 serving	1 serving
Spinach Salad with 2 T Low-fat Dressing	unlimited	unlimited

Snack:

Melon Cubes	1 cup	1 cup
Low-fat Swiss Cheese	1 oz.	1 oz.

Dinner:

Garlic Roasted Chicken	4 oz.	6 oz.
Cooked Bulgur	⅓ cup	⅔ cup
Pea Pods	1 cup	1 cup

Snack:

Low-fat Oatmeal Cookie	1 small	1 small
Fat-free Milk	1 cup	1 cup

Day 13	Women's Plan	Men's Plan

Breakfast:

Low-fat Vegetarian Sausage	2 links	3 links
Fresh Cherries	12	12
Whole-Wheat English Muffin	½	1

Lunch:

Turkey Salad made with light mayonnaise	½ cup	¾ cup
Cucumbers and Radishes	unlimited	unlimited
Pumpernickel Bread	1 slice	2 slices

Snack:

Raspberries	1 cup	1 cup
Light Vanilla Yogurt	1 cup	1 cup

Dinner:

Pan-Seared Trout with Pine Nuts and Pumpkin Seeds (see recipe)	1 serving	1 serving
Steamed Red-Skin Potato	½ cup	1 cup
Steamed Cauliflower	1 cup	1 cup

Snack:

Whole-Wheat Ginger Snaps	3 small	3 small
Fat-free Milk	1 cup	1 cup

Day 14	Women's Plan	Men's Plan

Breakfast:

Lean Turkey Bacon	2 slices	3 slices
Fresh Blueberries	¾ cup	¾ cup
Whole-Grain Oat Pancake	1	2
Sugar-free Syrup	2 Tbsp.	2 Tbsp.

Lunch:

Low-fat Shrimp Salad made with light mayo	½ cup	¾ cup
Avocado	⅛ medium	⅛ medium
Tomato	1 medium	1 medium
Pasta Salad with Fat-free Dressing	½ cup	1 cup

Snack:

Plum	2 medium	2 medium
String Cheese	1 oz.	1 oz.

Dinner:

Broiled Lean Lamb Chop	4 oz.	6 oz.
Curried Couscous	⅓ cup	⅔ cup
Steamed Yellow Squash	1 cup	1 cup

Snack:

Kiwi	1 large	1 large
Light Yogurt	1 cup	1 cup

Day 15	Women's Plan	Men's Plan

Breakfast:

Scrambled Egg Substitute	½ cup	1 cup
Cantaloupe Wedge	⅓ medium	⅓ medium
Rye Toast	1 slice	2 slices

Lunch:

Open-Faced Turkey Reuben (see recipe)	1	1

Snack:

Fresh Pineapple	¾ cup	¾ cup
Cottage Cheese	¼ cup	¼ cup

Dinner:

Stir-Fried Tofu	6 oz.	8 oz.
Basmati Rice	⅓ cup	⅔ cup
Red and Yellow Bell Peppers	1 cup	1 cup

Snack:

Peach Frozen Yogurt (see recipe)	1 serving	1 serving

Day 16	Women's Plan	Men's Plan

Breakfast:

Low-fat Granola	⅓ cup	⅔ cup
Fresh Blueberries	¾ cup	¾ cup
Light Vanilla Yogurt	1 cup	1 cup

Lunch:

Salmon Salad made with light mayo	½ cup	¾ cup
Butter-leaf Lettuce Salad with 2 T low-fat dressing	unlimited	unlimited
Wasa Crackers	2	4

Snack:

Nectarine	1	1
Low-fat Ricotta Cheese	¼ cup	¼ cup

Dinner:

Baked Chicken Breast	4 oz.	6 oz.
Herbed Wild Rice	½ cup	1 cup
French Cut Green Beans	1 cup	1 cup

Snack:

Orange	1	1
Fat-free Milk	1 cup	1 cup

Day 17	Women's Plan	Men's Plan

Breakfast:

Low-fat Muesli	½ cup	1 cup
Banana, 9"	½	½
Fat-free Milk	1 cup	1 cup

Lunch:

Lean Roast Beef	2 oz.	3 oz.
Coleslaw made with low-fat mayo	1 cup	1 cup
Pumpernickel Bread	1 slice	2 slices

Snack:

Dried Cranberries	2 Tbsp.	2 Tbsp.
Fat-free Yogurt	1 cup	1 cup

Dinner:

Turkey Tostados (see recipe)	1 serving	1 serving
Low-fat Grated Carrot Salad	1 cup	1 cup

Snack:

Kiwi	1 medium	1 medium
Cottage Cheese	¼ cup	¼ cup

Day 18	Women's Plan	Men's Plan

Breakfast:

Tropical Breakfast Smoothie (see recipe)	1 serving	1 serving

Lunch:

Crabmeat Salad made with light mayo	½ cup	¾ cup
Avocado	⅛ medium	⅛ medium
Sliced Tomato	1 medium	1 medium
Pasta Salad with 2 T fat-free dressing	½ cup	1 cup

Snack:

Nectarine	1	1
Low-fat Ricotta Cheese	¼ cup	¼ cup

Dinner:

Baked Pork or Veal Chop	4 oz.	6 oz.
Wild Rice and Mushroom Pilaf	½ cup	1 cup
Steamed Asparagus	1 cup	1 cup

Snack:

Pumpernickel Melba Crisp	5 oblong	5 oblong
Fat-free Milk	1 cup	1 cup

Day 19	Women's Plan	Men's Plan

Breakfast:

Scrambled Egg Substitute	½ cup	1 cup
Orange	1	1
Sourdough Toast	1 slice	2 slices

Lunch:

Tuna and White Bean Salad (see recipe)	1 serving	1 serving

Snack:

Tangerines	2	2
Light Yogurt	1 cup	1 cup

Dinner:

Lean Turkey Burger	4 oz.	6 oz.
Multigrain Roll	1	1½
Broccoli Salad with 2 T fat-free dressing	1 cup	1 cup

Snack:

Strawberry Shake made with Whey Protein mixed in water	1 scoop	1 scoop
Fresh Strawberries	1¼ cups	1¼ cups

Day 20	Women's Plan	Men's Plan

Breakfast:

Scrambled Egg Whites	3	4
Grapefruit	½	½
Oatmeal Toast	1 slice	2 slices

Lunch:

Lean Roast Beef	2 oz.	3 oz.
Lettuce and Tomato Slices	unlimited	unlimited
Whole-Grain Pita	½	1

Snack:

Blackberries	1 cup	1 cup
Fat-free Vanilla Yogurt	1 cup	1 cup

Dinner:

Broiled Flounder	4 oz.	6 oz.
Brown and Wild Rice Pilaf	⅓ cup	⅔ cup
Brussels Sprouts	1 cup	1 cup

Snack:

Oat Bran Pretzels	¾ oz.	¾ oz.
Fat-free Milk	1 cup	1 cup

Sample Menus for Weekends (more prep time required)

Day 21	Women's Plan	Men's Plan

Breakfast:

Lox, Eggs, and Onions (see recipe)	1 serving	1 serving

Pink Grapefruit	½	½
Pumpernickel Toast	1 slice	2 slices

Lunch:

Vegetable Quesadilla (see recipe)	1 serving	1 serving
Mixed Green Salad with 2 T low-fat dressing	unlimited	unlimited

Snack:

Blueberries	¾ cup	¾ cup
Cottage Cheese	¼ cup	½ cup

Dinner:

Beef Stew (see recipe)	1 serving	1 serving
Spinach Salad with 2 T low-fat dressing	unlimited	unlimited

Snack:

Chocolate Pudding (see recipe)	1 serving	1 serving

Day 22	Women's Plan	Men's Plan

Breakfast:

Fresh Berry and Yogurt Parfait (see recipe)	1 serving	1 serving

Lunch:

Cobb Salad (see recipe)	1 serving	1 serving
Sourdough Roll	1	1

Snack:

Apple	1 small	1 small
Low-fat String Cheese	1 oz.	1 oz.

Dinner:

Rainbow Trout with Pesto (see recipe)	1 serving	1 serving
Brown Rice	⅓ cup	⅔ cup
Steamed Broccoli	1 cup	1 cup

Snack:

Poached Pears (see recipe)	1 serving	1 serving

Day 23	Women's Plan	Men's Plan

Breakfast:

Maple Granola (see recipe)	1 serving	1½ servings
Fat-free Milk	1 cup	1 cup
Banana, 9"	½	½

Lunch:

Turkey Roll-Up (see recipe)	1 serving	1 serving
Romaine and Carrot Salad with 2 T low-fat dressing	unlimited	unlimited

Snack:

Fresh Raspberries	1 cup	1 cup
Plain Yogurt	1 cup	1 cup

Dinner:

Marinated Asian Beef Salad (see recipe)	1 serving	1 serving
Brown Rice	1/3 cup	2/3 cup

Snack:

Mango Custard (see recipe)	1 serving	1 serving

Day 24	Women's Plan	Men's Plan

Breakfast:

Soy Breeze (see recipe)	1 serving	1 serving

Lunch:

Mexican Black Bean and Salsa Salad (see recipe)	1 serving	1 serving

Snack:

Fresh Pineapple Chunks	3/4 cup	3/4 cup
Low-fat Ricotta Cheese	1/4 cup	1/2 cup

Dinner:

Mussels Marinara (see recipe)	1 serving	1 serving
Pasta cooked al dente	1/2 cup	1 cup
Steamed Zucchini	1 cup	1 cup

Snack:

Peanut Butter Cookie (see recipe)	1	1

Day 25	Women's Plan	Men's Plan

Breakfast:

Provencal Style Frittata (see recipe)	1 serving	1 serving
Cantaloupe Cubes	1 cup	1 cup

Lunch:

Salmon Corn Chowder (see recipe)	1 serving	1 serving
Spinach and Mushroom Salad with 2 T low-fat dressing	unlimited	unlimited
Multigrain Roll	1	1

Snack:

Pear	1 small	1 small
Fat-free Milk	1 cup	1 cup

Dinner:

Southwestern Meatloaf (see recipe)	1 serving	1 serving
Barley	⅓ cup	⅔ cup
Steamed Asparagus	1 cup	1 cup

Snack:

Chocolate-Covered Strawberries (see recipe)	1 serving	1 serving

Day 26	Women's Plan	Men's Plan

Breakfast:

Banana Chocolate Chip Muffin	1	1
Light Vanilla Yogurt	1 cup	1 cup

Lunch:

Baked Tofu Chef's Salad (see recipe)	1 serving	1 serving
Rye Roll	none	1 small

Snack:

Honeydew Cubes	1 cup	1 cup
Low-fat Swiss Cheese	1 oz.	1 oz.

Dinner:

Tilapia with Honey Mustard Sauce (see recipe)	1 serving	1 serving
Couscous	⅓ cup	⅔ cup
Stir-fried Snow Peas and Red Bell Peppers	1 cup	1 cup

Snack:

Peach and Blueberry Crisp (see recipe)	1 serving	1 serving

Day 27	Women's Plan	Men's Plan

Breakfast:

Southwest Egg Scramble (see recipe)	1 serving	1 serving
Orange	1	1

Lunch:

Vegetable Miso Soup (see recipe)	1 serving	1 serving
Tossed Green Salad with 2 T low-fat dressing	unlimited	unlimited

Snack:		
Fresh Cherries	12	12
Vanilla Yogurt	1 cup	1 cup
Dinner:		
Turkey London Broil (see recipe)	4 oz.	6 oz.
Herbed Wild Rice	½ cup	1 cup
Grilled Eggplant	1 cup	1 cup
Snack:		
Baked Fruit Alaska (see recipe)	1 serving	1 serving

Day 28	Women's Plan	Men's Plan
Breakfast:		
Cheese Omelet with Salsa (see recipe)	1 serving	1 serving
Honeydew Melon Wedge	⅛ medium	⅛ medium
Lunch:		
Antipasto Salad with Tuna (see recipe)	1 serving	1 serving
Pumpernickel Roll	none	1
Snack:		
Mango	½ medium	½ medium
Plain Yogurt	1 cup	1 cup
Dinner:		
Thai Chicken with Broccoli (see recipe)	1 serving	1 serving
Steamed Brown Rice	⅓ cup	⅔ cup
Snack:		
Blueberry Cheesecake (see recipe)	1 serving	1 serving

NutriSystem Nourish Prepared Foods Meal Plan

This plan features the new NutriSystem Nourish prepared foods that you purchase from NutriSystem and adds in fresh fruits, vegetables, and salads. This plan works best for those who lead busy lives and want convenience without sacrificing taste. You simply choose your breakfast, lunch, and dinner entrées plus a dessert for each day and follow the menu plan outlined to start losing weight. All the healthy nutrition, taste, and portions are built in—there's no weighing, measuring or counting points. You don't need to think about monitoring your low-glycemic carbohydrates, fats, or proteins; the NutriSystem Nourish foods do that for you on this plan. Just choose your foods and start losing weight.

A sample menu that illustrates how the new NutriSystem Nourish foods would fit into your daily meal plan is included here. The foods are simply representative of the nearly 100 great-tasting NutriSystem items (see foods list to follow) and countless grocery food additions you can include to complete your Prepared Foods Meal Plan.

Prepared Foods Meal Plan—Sample Menu

	Women's Plan	Men's Plan
Breakfast:		
NutriSystem Breakfast Entrée	Scrambled Eggs with Vegetables	Scrambled Eggs with Vegetables
Fruit Serving	1 cup Cantaloupe Cubes	1 cup Cantaloupe Cubes
Dairy Serving	Fat-free Milk (1 cup)	Fat-free Milk (1 cup)
Grain/Bread Serving	None	1 slice Pumpernickel Toast
Lunch:		
NutriSystem Lunch Entrée	Hearty Minestrone Soup	Hearty Minestrone Soup
Salad Vegetables	Mixed Greens, Mushrooms, and Cucumbers	Mixed Greens, Mushrooms, and Cucumbers
NutriSystem Low-fat Salad Dressing	Italian Dressing (2 Tbsp.)	Italian Dressing (2 Tbsp.)
Dairy Serving	Light Yogurt (1 cup)	Light Yogurt (1 cup)
Grain/Bread Serving	none	1 Multigrain Roll
Snack:		
Dairy Serving	Cottage Cheese (¼ cup)	Cottage Cheese (¼ cup)
Fruit Serving	Raspberries (1 cup)	Raspberries (1 cup)
Dinner:		
NutriSystem Dinner Entrée	BBQ Beef with Rice and Beans	BBQ Beef with Rice and Beans
Vegetable Serving	Green Beans (1 cup)	Green Beans (1 cup)
Salad or Fruit Serving	Spinach Salad	Spinach Salad
Fat Serving	Olive Oil (1 tsp.)	Olive Oil (2 tsp.)
Grain/Bread Serving	none	Corn (½ cup)
Snack:		
NutriSystem Dessert	Mochaccino Dessert Bar	Mochaccino Dessert Bar

NutriSystem Nourish Prepared Foods List

NutriSystem is proud to introduce its new line of foods! There are almost a hundred great-tasting options for you to choose from, each designed to have a low glycemic index value and optimal amounts of protein, fats, and fiber and to fit into the new NutriSystem Nourish program.

NutriSystem Nourish Breakfast Entrées

Scrambled Eggs

Scrambled Eggs with Cheddar Cheese

Scrambled Eggs with Peppers and Mushrooms

Oatmeal

Apple Cinnamon Oatmeal

NutriCinnamon Squares Cereal

NutriCoconut O's Cereal

NutriFrosted Crunch Cereal

NutriFlakes Cereal

Low-Fat Granola

Frosted Oats Cereal

Mini Frosted Shredded Wheat Cereal

Chocolate Chip Granola Bar

Apple Granola Bar

Cranberry Granola Bar

Lemon Poppyseed Muffin

Banana Spice Muffin

Blueberry Bran Muffin

NutriSystem Nourish Lunch Entrées

Bean and Ham Soup

Black Beans and Rice

Blueberry Low-Fat Yogurt

Chicken Cacciatore

Chicken Noodle Soup

Chicken Salad

Cream of Broccoli Soup

Fettuccini Alfredo with Vegetables and Mushrooms

Sliced Ham with Whole Wheat Deli Roll

Tomato Sauce & Meatballs with Whole Wheat Roll

Hearty Minestrone Soup

Noodles with Chicken and Vegetables

Pasta Parmesan with Broccoli

Pasta Salad with Ham

Pasta with Beef

Spicy Oriental Noodles with Vegetables and Peanuts

Strawberry Low-Fat Yogurt

Sweet & Sour Chicken

Tex-Mex Rice and Beans

Tuna Salad

Turkey Hot Dog with Whole Wheat Deli Roll

Vegetable Beef Soup

Vegetarian Pasta Salad

Vegetarian Sloppy Joe with Whole Wheat Roll

NutriSystem Nourish Dinner Entrées

BBQ Sauce with White Chicken Fillet with Whole Wheat Roll

BBQ Sauce over Beef, Beans, and Rice

Beef and Mushroom Gravy with Rice

Beef Stroganoff with Noodles

Beef Tacos

Beef with Peppercorn Sauce and Vegetables

Burgundy Sauce and Beef with Rice

Cheese and Spinach Ravioli with Meat Sauce

Chicken Breast Patty with Whole Wheat Roll

Chicken Pasta Parmesan

Chicken Primavera with Pasta

Chicken with Almonds, Rice and Vegetables

Chili with Beans

Fillet of Fish with Lemon Butter Sauce and Wild Rice

Cheeseburger with Whole Wheat Roll

Hamburger with Whole Wheat Roll

Holiday Turkey Breast with Diced Potatoes and Gravy

Green Pepper Steak with Rice

Hearty Beef Stew

Homestyle Chicken Noodles with Gravy

Macaroni with Cheese and Beef

Mushroom Gravy over Salisbury Steak and Rice

Orange Beef with Noodles

Oriental Style Chicken with Rice and Lemon Ginger Sauce

Polynesian Style Pork

Pot Roast Gravy over Beef, Potatoes, and Carrots

Rotini with Meatballs and Tomato Sauce

Seafood Newburg

Sliced Roast Beef in Gravy with Whole Wheat Roll

Spicy Oriental Style Chicken with Vegetables and Rice

Teriyaki Sauce and Beef with Rice

Thin Crust Pizza with Cheese

Thin Crust Pizza with Peppers and Mushrooms

Three Cheese Pasta with Chicken

Vegetable Lasagna with Meat Sauce

Zesty Cajun Style Chicken with Wild Rice

NutriSystem Nourish Desserts and Snacks

Almond Pistachio Biscotti

Amaretto Coffee

Apple Cinnamon Soy Chips

BBQ Soy Chips

Blueberry Lemon Dessert Bar

Cappuccino Coffee

Chocolate Macadamia Nut Biscotti

Chocolate Mochaccino Dessert
  Bar
Chocolate Peanut Butter Dessert
  Bar
Chocolate Pudding
Chocolate Shake
Hot Cocoa

Mint Hot Cocoa
Mocha Shake
NutriCrunch Chocolates
Sour Cream and Onion Soy
  Chips
Vanilla Pudding
White Cheddar Soy Chips

If you have any questions regarding which plan may suit you best, call a NutriSystem counselor at 1-800-321-THIN, or log on to the NutriSystem Web site at www.nutrisystem.com for more information.

PART THREE

Nourishing Movement

6

Move It to Lose It
You Choose: Xercise or Xtra Size?

Exercise is a key ingredient to any weight-loss effort. Movement is a core element of any healthy lifestyle. Move it or you won't lose it. Exercise has been proven to help people lose weight and keep it off. Period.

Some of you out there may not like hearing that. And some of you may be tempted to let it go in one ear and right out the other. But please, do pay attention to this. It's good news: *Exercise will help you reach your weight-loss goal.* It will make you feel healthier and stronger and will give you the additional motivation to stick to the NutriSystem Nourish plan. I realize that for many people getting regular exercise not only seems like a daunting task but also brings up a load of historical baggage from past performances that's hard to overcome. You may have some history with movement that is less than positive—a gym class failed, an exercise goal missed, an embarrassing experience at the health club or something that happened when you were young. If you are carrying around that kind of baggage, it's painful and it does nothing to serve your present good or goals for the future. My advice is to start immediately and optimistically commit to changing your thinking—maybe even head back to Chapter 3 and restructure your mindset about exercise. Call up that old gym teacher; burn that old workout gear—do whatever you need to do to address whatever may be holding you back from opening yourself up to exercise and movement—but do it now. Strive to move on. Because, really, you simply must move.

This program is about more than just a "diet"; this is about creating a lifestyle in which you can maintain a healthy weight for the long term, and to do so, that lifestyle must include regular exercise. Deep down, you already know that.

Aside from providing you with specific exercise routines that are easy to do and simple to follow, as outlined in the next chapter, the NutriSystem Nourish program itself allows you time and space to incorporate exercise into your life. And because you'll be working at nourishing all parts of your self—body and mind—exercise will seem like a natural progression and part of the program.

The fitness element that I've developed to go along with the nutritional part of the NutriSystem Nourish program is time sensitive, can be done at home, and can be done without a major investment in any big fitness equipment. It was designed with you in mind—the busy person, looking for ways simply to fit exercise into a hectic schedule. Don't jump ahead and check out the routines just yet. I want to take some time in this chapter to explain to you why exercising is so important and to run down in more detail some of your fitness options. I'm going to outline the who, what, when, where, why, and how much of exercise, filling you in on the best way to incorporate fitness into your life.

> The biggest risk to exercise is not starting.
>
> —The American College of Sports Medicine

Why Should I Exercise?

Have you ever noticed how good you feel after a healthy walk, an inspired dance, or a refreshing swim? Or how you come alive during a backyard game of catch or football with your kids, nieces, or nephews? It's a different kind of awareness, a different kind of awake. Your entire being feels more alive, more creative, more possible.

Exercise is a key link to achieving optimum wellness. When you exercise, you will absolutely perform at a higher, more complete level in every aspect of your life. When we witness our self-discipline coming through for us and creating daily invigorating movement, we set a tone for our day and our entire life that leads to personal, professional, and spiritual excellence.

Most of us naturally associate exercise with its physical benefits, such as less fat, more muscle, better circulation, improved heart function, and even looking better. We've been taught since we were young that exercise and good health go hand in hand, but why?

Exercise initiates a cascade of chemical events that enliven your body and your whole being. Exercise enhances the transport of oxygen and nutrients into the cells. It also helps your body remove waste and improve general circulation. It's key to your weight-loss program because it helps to counter the reduction in basal metabolic rate (BMR) that often accompanies simply dieting alone without fitness. Exercise increases the BMR for an extended period of time following your movement period—it gets your metabolism moving. Exercise also helps decrease your appetite by increasing levels of naturally occurring satisfaction chemicals in your body. And since muscle is the primary burner of fat calories, building muscle through exercise will increase your fat-burning efficiency. Movement maximizes your natural affinity to burn fat.

> That which is used develops. That which is not, wastes away.
>
> —Hippocrates

Beyond just the physical benefits of exercise, there is more and more exciting evidence linking it to emotional well-being, which is also a precursor to weight-loss success. No question about it, regular exercise promotes happiness, self-esteem, and optimism. When we exercise, our bodies naturally produce chemicals that counter negative feelings and emotions such as depression and anxiety. Vigorous exercise, even for short periods of time, causes blood endorphin levels to rise far above their normal levels for several hours, contributing to improved mood and a sense of well-being.

Norepinephrine is a brain chemical that helps to promote feelings of energy, confidence, and motivation. Release of this chemical happens through exercise, which means through movement you can literally create it whenever you need it. It can help to squash the hormones that make you feel like moving right to the kitchen to feed your stress!

Norepinephrine can be a critical tool for you to use when fighting your vulnerability windows, too. Most of us have windows during the day when we are more vulnerable to making less-than-wonderful choices. Take notice as to what and when those windows are for you and what you are doing at that time of vulnerability. You may notice a trend. Perhaps you are either sitting down and stressing or sitting down after stressing. Both of these scenarios can promote the same outcome of eating foods that are not great for you or your goals.

Exercise causes a whole landslide of positive chemical effects in the body and mind. But from what I've seen and experienced, the proverbial psychological high that you feel during and after exercise can most likely be attributed to one overriding factor: having achieved your goal. Truly. A sense of accomplishment cannot be underrated, and the greater the challenge of the exercise, the greater your sense of achievement will be.

Studies have shown that exercisers feel more in charge of their lives. And having a proactive sense of yourself certainly can play a huge part in better managing your stress, attending to important physical, emotional, and spiritual needs, and supporting overall satisfaction in all areas of your life. People who exercise regularly have a better opportunity to experience the life that they desire. On the flip side, research also indicates that many adults who choose not to include exercise in their lives have a higher incidence of depression, anxiety, general moodiness, and issues surrounding fatigue.

> "I am not an exerciser. I do not exercise!" I clearly remember telling Dr. James that when I first consulted him for weight loss. "'No problem," he replied, and asked me to tell him what activities I do all day long. I proceeded to walk him through my busy life. He showed me, from a new perspective, that I could exercise. In the beginning, I just started to give a little extra effort to everyday activities, and I started to feel stronger. My intention began to grow. I started seeing all kinds of new ways to approach my life duties and responsibilities. I began to see them as a way to do something for myself—I saw myself as more physical, more alive. Today, I find myself walking whenever I can, and I am more active in every area in my life. I still kid Dr. James that I do not exercise, but I sure am moving a lot more! —Celeste, 54

Let's face it—everyone knows that they should exercise. Yet we find time for plenty of excuses, like, "But I don't enjoy exercise," or, "But I'm too tired." Remember our "But" Reduction exercise? To begin with, barring some serious physical or medical condition, there really is no excuse for not exercising, but you do need to want to do it. While you can't view exercise as an option, you can definitely strive to make it as enjoyable as possible. It should be! The results should be enjoyable, too. Exercise cannot be an "I'll try to fit it in" thing in your life. It needs to be a priority at the top of your to-you list.

Why exercise? Because you deserve it. And without it, your weight-loss efforts and your spirit will suffer. By exercising, you'll discover the feeling of being able to do, to create, and to make life happen. Through invigorating and enjoyable exercise, your physical transition will begin and changes will arise from the inside out.

A Day in the Life of NutriSystem Nourish

Joe follows the Prepared Foods Meal Plan 100 percent for his weight loss program.

Joe is a 41-year-old bachelor trying to slim down and balance his life. It's Wednesday, and by 6 A.M., he's showered, dressed, and off to work. He downs his daily multivitamin with a glass of fat-free milk and heads out the door with a NutriSystem Chocolate Chip Granola Bar and an orange in hand. By noon, he's done at least three deep breathing exercises during twice as many stressful meetings, and he takes off for the gym to get his weight-lifting workout in. Energized, he returns to his office and prepares his NutriSystem Black Beans and Rice, enjoying it along with the salad and low-fat yogurt that he picked up at the convenience store on the way.

Before his 3:30 meeting, Joe grabs two cans of V-8 from the vending machine and drinks them while getting the lowdown on corporate earnings. At 6:30 P. M., he's still at his desk and heads to the microwave once again to heat up some NutriSystem Cheese and Spinach Ravioli with Meat Sauce. He eats that, along with what's left of his salad from lunch, some carrot sticks he had thrown in his cooler pack, and half of a leftover low-fat muffin he snagged from the break room earlier in the day. By 8 P.M., Joe is finally home, decompressing, and considering some relaxing plans for the weekend while munching on NutriCrunch Chocolates.

It's been another great day on the NutriSystem Nourish program for Joe.

Who Should Be Exercising?

How many of you have ever said, "Oh, I'm just too old to start exercising," or, "Oh, I'm just too achy and I think exercise would do me in. I haven't moved around like that since I was a kid. I think I'd have a heart attack if I did that now." The truth is, you're probably more likely to have that heart attack if you *don't* start exercising now!

Is it ever too late to begin exercising? No way! You can always begin a regular exercise program or at least walking and moving and experience wondrous results physically and emotionally. Your body will adapt well to an exercise program because it craves it, and it will begin delivering strength through increased muscle tone and mental clarity through an increased release of hormones and endorphins no matter what your age.

Listen to this compelling news. Regular exercise slows the aging process, no matter when you begin. Scientists use various tests to grade the aging process and investigate these criteria:

- Aerobic capacity
- Basal metabolic rate
- Blood pressure
- Blood sugar tolerance
- Body fat
- Body temperature regulation
- Bone density
- Cholesterol levels
- Lean body mass
- Overall strength

And they've found that no matter what your age, every one of these tests can be influenced for the better. Once developed, exercise is a habit that will actually help you grow physiologically younger instead of older.

Think of it this way: exercise is much like a pension plan—the more you contribute now, the better your quality of life will be later. It's never too late to begin a program of strengthening yourself physically, mentally, and emotionally. You can look great and feel great starting right now. So stretch yourself, regardless of your age or your size.

Maybe you've noticed that most exercise programs and equipment are not made for larger-size people. Or maybe you once purchased a gym membership, showed up, felt uncomfortable, left, and never went back. Perhaps you have a basement full of unused exercise equipment gathering dust. I do not know your personal story, but I do know this: the NutriSystem Nourish exercise plan is doable for you. I created this plan to be different. No matter what your story, your size, your fitness level or lack thereof, you will find this program more than within your capabilities, I promise. My wish is that you will find it encouraging and fun. But most importantly, I know that by incorporating this fitness plan into your life, you will have success with the entire weight-loss program and enjoy your results.

With the NutriSystem Nourish program for movement, you will feel better right away. Right from the beginning, you will see that you can have success, and through that initial success your spirit, confidence, and conviction will soar. You'll learn to trust and embrace the understanding that you really do have the ability to move and to move well. You can do this. You can be active. It's not about having to perform exercises that were designed for someone more mobile than you; in fact, you can perform many of this plan's movements without even having to get into any uncomfortable or compromising positions. Ours is a simple, practical approach to fitness.

How Much and How Often Should I Exercise?

Often we hear all kinds of conflicting information on how much or how often we should exercise. Remember, it is not about throwing yourself into an area where you come up feeling like you sacrificed 20 minutes for the sake of health—that's the wrong mentality. This process can and should be enjoyed.

How much time should you dedicate to your program? The answer lies in your envisioned outcome. For optimal health, most people need to burn roughly 300 calories daily. This is roughly equivalent to 40 to 45 minutes of swimming (slowly), 45 minutes to an hour of walking, or about 50 minutes of cycling (10 mph). If you only have a 30-minute window, you may choose to cross-train instead (doing a combination of activities in smaller increments of time), in order to get an efficient, well-rounded workout. This could be as simple as 10 minutes of walking or jogging, 10 minutes on a bike, and 10 minutes of weight training each day. In one-half hour, you will improve your heart function, strengthen your bones, and improve your emotional outlook for the entire day, not to mention encourage more and more weight loss.

Add It Up

Don't limit yourself to just one aerobic exercise. Experiment with different activities and don't be afraid to combine more than one aerobic activity in one exercise session. For example:

- 10 minutes brisk walking plus 10 minutes stationary bike
- 20 minutes swimming plus 10 minutes stair climber
- 15 minutes jogging plus 10 minutes jumping rope
- 10 minutes rowing machine plus 15 minutes treadmill

At a minimum, I recommend that you set a goal of moving at least 20 minutes each day, and allow for flexibility. If you have two 10-minute windows on a given day and not a total of 20 minutes altogether, then go for the two 10-minute sessions and you'll still get great results. Movement is about freedom, so please realize that each day you have within you the ability to be creative and flexible and choose what works best for you. Move beyond the less-than-empowering history of how exercise must be done with a lot of physical and emotional heaviness, and consider instead how movement can be experienced with lightness and creativity.

Many of my patients ask me how hard they should be exercising. Should they be struggling a lot or should there be any pain? The answer is no. You do not need to experience pain for exercise to be effective. The old adage "No pain, no gain" is dead and gone, and we now know that any and all movement is beneficial and that it's never good to work your body so hard that you are too sore to follow through with your plan during the next session. Allow your body's wisdom to dictate the pace and intensity of your exercise. You will notice that on some days you really feel like going for it and other days it feels like just getting through it is a battle. That's okay and very normal. Just don't overdo it, especially in the beginning, or you'll set yourself up for disappointment.

But be wary of this: a surefire way to kill any exercise program before it even really starts is to begin it so enthusiastically that your body just can't keep up. You know, like heading out for a 6-mile hike through the woods when you haven't taken a walk in 10 years. Unfortunately, I see this happen time and time again. While I admire the zeal, inspiration, and drive, you must begin in moderation and start out slowly. Whatever exercise you choose, set a reasonable pace for you and stick with it. You can't live life in a day, nor can you create lifelong fitness in one. Most injuries from exercise happen to the weekend warriors—a population that does not warm up but still approaches a sport full throttle and ultimately ends up in pain. This is not what you want.

Be sure to consult your physician for evaluation and clearance before beginning any new exercise program.

Ideally you should choose to move daily, and you should look forward to it as an opportunity to lift your spirit, support your weight-loss efforts, and optimize your health. It really will feel good, and it can change your perspective on everything.

Exercise Tips

- Keep a pair of light weights (5 to 10 pounds each) in a handy place like your bedroom, where you will be reminded of your fitness goals.
- When you are watching television, do 15 push-ups and 15 abdominal crunches during each set of commercial breaks.
- Know that you are making a big difference in your life and that you are also setting a positive example for your children and your friends.
- Place exercise reminder notes on your computer, telephone, and alarm clock—at home and at the office—wherever you are likely to see them.

When Should I Exercise?

Would you consider waking up 30 minutes earlier if it meant you would sleep better at night, focus better during the day, burn more calories, and jumpstart your metabolism?

Most people who engage in a consistent fitness program exercise in the morning. And from my own experience, both personally and clinically, I've found that morning exercise regimes tend to be more successful for longer periods of time than those done later in the day. It makes sense. In the morning hours, when we plan ahead, our time is less likely to be disturbed. As our day progresses, things tend to come up—unplanned obstacles to our self-care. In the morning you can get your exercise in before anything can rock your schedule.

When you exercise early in the morning, it jumpstarts your metabolism and keeps it elevated for hours—sometimes up to 24 hours. How's that for fat-burning power? When you exercise at about the same time every morning and ideally wake up at about the same time on a regular basis, your body's endocrine system and circadian rhythms adjust to that, and physiologically your body reaps the rewards. In time, even hours prior to your waking up, your body will start to prepare for exercise because it knows what's about to happen and it has adjusted to doing the same thing every day. This adds to the ease with which you'll approach your exercise.

If you are worried about losing that half hour or so of sleep, know that research demonstrates that people who exercise regularly have a higher quality of sleep and require less sleep, anyway. You'll be reaping the fringe benefits of having set an awesome tone for the day and you'll experience increased energy, improved mood, and a stronger sense of confidence and optimism—all from those 30 minutes.

However, if you're not a morning person or if you're too busy shuffling off kids or spouses or yourself in the morning to focus on exercise, please don't dismay. Again, when it comes to exercise, the key thing is that you do it and that you do it consistently. Maybe your exercise time falls during your lunch hour. Or maybe hitting the health club on your way home from work fits perfectly into your lifestyle. That's great, too. Just find something that works for you and stick with it.

Breaking Up Is Easy to Do

So you say that you don't have 20 or 30 minutes to exercise. No problem! You can break up your exercise time and piece together these moves to move you toward your goal:

- Take the stairs instead of the escalator or elevator.
- Park in the farthest rather than the closest spot when shopping.
- Walk to your favorite store.
- Practice contracting, then relaxing the muscles of your belly, butt, thighs, calves, and arms while you drive, commute by train or subway, or sit and watch TV.

Every day, try to inspire and challenge yourself to find new ways and places to move!

What Exercise Should I Do?

The best exercise for burning fat, increasing health, and improving your overall well-being is a combination of movements: the blending of aerobic, strength, and flexibility exercises will ensure that you are getting the highest yield from your investment.

However, with all the different types of exercise programs, classes, equipment, and videos, it is often overwhelming to choose what to do. To tell you the truth, though, most exercise works when you do it habitually, so when I am asked which exercise is best for overall health and well-being, I simply reply, "The one that you will do consistently!"

In much the same way that eating one healthy meal will not give you lifelong dietary health, one solid exercise session will not give you sustained physical wellness, but an ongoing habit of it will. With any successful exercise program, consistency is the key to lasting health. So when choosing the form of exercise you desire, you need to choose something that you believe you can stick with. That's why the variety of cross-training—combining various exercises such as running followed by biking, or combining yoga practice with weight training or any of your other favorite exercises to create a total workout—appeals to so many. Its variety is the spice of many lives, and it can keep fitness from losing its luster.

Metabolic Minutes

Here are some exercises you can do around the house when you have a few minutes:

Kitchen Moves
- Do modified push-ups from the countertop or refrigerator.
- Extend a can of soup or pet food and do arm curls while you wait for the water to boil, oven to preheat, or microwave to sound off.
- Do modified squats from your kitchen chairs.

Living Room Moves
- Dance or walk in place during commercial breaks.
- Alternate one-leg lunges from the floor or coffee table.
- Do seated torso twists from the sofa or chair.

Bedroom Moves
- Lying on the floor or on the bed, alternate knee-to-chest stretches.
- Do side leg lifts from your dresser or bedpost support.
- Do supported squats from your bedroom wall.

Bathroom Moves
- Do modified squats from your toilet seat while brushing your teeth.

But before you begin anything, make an honest assessment of yourself and your goals. Ask yourself these questions: What is my desired outcome? How much time can I commit to regular exercise? And remember, your goal should always be personal excellence, and not perfection. Don't set yourself up for failure. Begin where you are and achieve what you can achieve. I suggest you begin realistically. Map out 1 month of your intended program, scheduling the time and type of exercise you will engage in each day.

In the next chapter, you'll find a complete 4-week workout routine that you can follow as your fitness plan. There are guidelines for those who are beginners, intermediate, or advanced exercisers. I've included everything from stretching and warm-up exercises to aerobic activities and weight training, and you'll see I've broken everything down specifically and have shown examples of how to do the moves. These workouts will guide you, step by step, through each day of your program.

You'll also see that within the plan I leave you some options. You'll always have the freedom to choose which kind of exercises to incorporate into your own individual plan (walking, running, jumping rope, treadmill, etc.) so that it can work for you. And that goes for the strength training routines from which you can choose and the relaxation elements, too. In my opinion, it's all about mixing it up so that the body doesn't lull itself into complacency. This is your exercise program and it needs to work for you.

Walk This Way

Have you ever noticed how a walk can change the state of things around and inside of you? Thoreau referred to a walk in the morning as "a blessing for the whole day." He was right. Walking offers many benefits both physically and mentally, not to mention that it can be done anytime, anywhere. That's why I advise patients to schedule a walk every day. You don't necessarily have to go out for hours at a time. Studies show that walking as little as 2 miles per day—for less than half an hour—is a superior exercise in terms of boosting metabolism and burning fat. It's actually better than if you were to run or jog the same distance. Walking takes longer, which actually encourages a stronger rise in metabolism. Since your caloric burn comes during the time after exercise, in the 24-hour period following a walk your body responds by burning all day, therefore burning more efficiently.

Here is a key: *walk every day.*

When it comes to heart-healthy exercise, many of us have the image of knock-down, drag-out, heavy-duty programs and cardio routines. However, research has found that simply walking 30 minutes daily at a brisk pace has a profound effect on reducing the incidence of heart disease. This low-tech, no-equipment-necessary method of exercise has proven itself. The *New England Journal of Medicine* reported a Boston study that showed walking 3 or more hours a week cut the threat of heart disease in women by 30 percent, and when increased to 5 or more hours per week, the risk of heart disease decreased more than 40 percent.

In Japan, there's a program called 10,000 steps a day. Its goal is simple—to encourage people to take 10,000 or more steps daily. While this may seem like a tall order, most sedentary loungers log at least 2,000 to 4,000 steps daily, and an average busy woman will log between 5,000 and 6,000 steps daily. By simply taking an additional 30-minute brisk walk, you can achieve 10,000 steps.

Other ways to create steps may include taking the stairs, taking a walk during your lunch break or after dinner, doing a walk-in-place program during TV commercials, or taking the parking space farthest away from the door. And because walking promotes clearer and more optimistic thinking, try this: when you're experiencing conflict, crisis, or an overwhelming feeling of powerlessness, change your venue and take a walk.

> ### Walk It Off
>
> Here is an exercise that has done wonders for many of my clients and their families.
>
> Often we experience considerable stress on our way home from work. A long day, traffic, and low blood sugar can create a less-than-open and unfriendly mood for you as you arrive home to be with your family. When you're in this situation, try this:
>
> When you arrive home, take a walk around the block, the yard, or down the street before going inside. Notice how you are after the brief exercise. The outcome is clear and compelling: motion creates a positive state of emotion that will increase your ability to be the person you want to be.

The Exercise Ball

You've probably seen some kind of big exercise ball recently, whether you know it or not. It looks like the "hippity hop" thing that you played with in childhood—minus the handles. These exercise balls are everywhere—at the gym, the office, in people's homes—and that's probably because just about everyone can benefit from "getting on the ball."

For starters, just sitting on the ball can lead to increased range of movement and improved balance, because while sitting on it, your body must make constant small adjustments to keep you balanced. These small adjustments improve circulation to the disks in your spine and can strengthen your back muscles. Gentle bouncing on the ball will encourage you to sit with the correct posture and help strengthen your postural muscles. If you take it one step further and lift one leg up a few inches from the floor, you'll notice it is more difficult to balance and you will begin to further engage the core stability muscles of your abdomen and spine.

Exercise balls are generally squishy and comfortable to sit on. They are sized according to height and you can buy them at almost any sporting goods store or even at some department stores. When choosing one for yourself, make sure you get the right size.

If you are shorter than 5'3"	55 cm ball
If you are between 5'3" and 5'6"	65 cm ball
If you are taller than 5'6"	75 cm ball

The balls have a high weight tolerance, so they are very strong and often come with their own pump, instruction booklet, and even sample exercise routines and videos. The balls themselves run around $15 to $30. Depending on what else is included in the package, the cost can go up from there.

While initially they may seem awkward or cumbersome to use, these balls are actually a great companion at the home or office, especially if you tend to sit in front of a computer all day. I incorporate the use of the ball into my workout routine whenever I can because of the toning and balancing element that it adds.

Please Weight

When I say weight lifting, do you envision images of muscle heads on Venice beach or scary-looking women on muscle magazine covers? If so, try to allow yourself to transcend these visions and open yourself to a new picture of balance, strength, and well being through strength-training.

Today's strength trainer looks like the actresses on TV or the executive in your boardroom, or the everyday people you see in the grocery store. The true story is that training with weights does not have to result in developing big muscles or matching attitudes, but it can encourage great muscle tone with radiant health. Best of all, you begin to notice improvement in strength and shape in just a few weeks or months with only a modest time commitment.

Resistance and strength training can contribute immensely to overall health and fitness. They help to improve your endurance, increase metabolism, support weight loss and the healthy management of weight, and for those struggling with osteoporosis, strength training increases bone mass.

Weight lifting also stimulates the release of human growth hormone (HGH), which in turn promotes an increased burning of fat. HGH is your body's most powerful fat-burning hormone and will work for you all night long. It is released at night while you sleep, so if you are not sleeping, you are not getting your support of HGH.

Why Weight?

- Weight training raises your resting metabolism. This causes you to burn more calories 24 hours a day (even while you're asleep).
- Weight training inspires greater energy and brightens your mood.
- Weight training strengthens your bones, reducing your risk of developing osteoporosis.
- Weight training strengthens your muscles, which looks great on you.
- Weight training makes you strong, and strength increases your self-esteem and self-confidence.
- Weight training can help lower your blood pressure.
- Weight training decreases your risk of developing adult-onset diabetes.
- Weight training improves the functioning of your immune system.
- Weight training improves your balance and coordination.

Strength training is empowering because you will see and feel results. To me, moving weights is a metaphor for moving obstacles in life. With every repetition it's like you are moving a personal challenge. Life offers resistance and sometimes you may want to give up and settle for mediocrity. But you won't! Your weight training can set the tone for your life's direction. When facing obstacles and adversity, you'll know that you do have the means and strength to move this weight.

Another great thing about weight training is that you can participate at any age. Studies show that no matter when you begin, consistent weight training can produce great benefits. A group of ten 90-year-old people who used canes or walkers began a resistance and strength training program. In just 5 weeks, all showed substantial strength gains, with seven of the ten participants eventually walking without the use of their canes or walkers. It's truly inspiring to know no matter what your past or how long of a past you have, every day holds a new opportunity to move toward well-being.

When it comes to weight lifting, I'm often asked which I think is better: free weights or the weight machines you find at health clubs. And I usually answer neither. I just encourage people to do one or the other (or both!) and to participate in weight training consistently.

If you have access to a fitness center where there are a lot of weight machines, go ahead and schedule a few sessions with a qualified personal trainer so that you learn proper techniques on those. Either option is great. Just choose what works best for you.

I am also a big fan of traditional exercises like push-ups, pull-ups, chin-ups, dips, and sit-ups. To this day, they remain some of the most effective exercises out there. So please don't use the "I can't afford the equipment" excuse. You don't need expensive, state-of-the-art gym equipment to get the results of strength training. Use your body weight to your advantage. If you can do one push-up now, imagine how many you will do when you are pushing up a lighter body!

Whatever you choose to do, approach weight training sensibly. Be clear of your goals. Be methodological in your plans. If you're using heavy weights, use a spotter when appropriate and never sacrifice proper form for a heavier weight. Allow your muscles to recover after working them by rotating your muscle groups and waiting a minimum of 2 days before working out the same muscle group again. And remember, always warm up with stretching and lighter weights before diving in!

Daily Moving

Weight-loss success and maintenance can be achieved by incorporating fitness into your daily life. You need to move it to lose it, and this program will help you.

The beauty of the NutriSystem Nourish program and its fitness component is that your exercise plan will not be an island all by itself—it's completely surrounded by invigorating foods, a balanced meal plan, and tools for maintaining your focus and motivation. Exercise was built right into the total plan. We provide you with a step-by-step guide to movement and fitness so that you can complete the total weight-loss picture and achieve maximum results. This is a core difference between the NutriSystem Nourish program and other weight-loss programs. This program offers an integrated approach to incorporating exercise into your life and fosters physical well-being in the context of your whole life. It's practical, reasonable, and very doable, and you'll get results if you follow it.

The toughest obstacle to overcome when starting any regular exercise program can be the first 3 to 6 weeks when your body, your habits, and your old desires for comfort are still trying to hang on. Prepare yourself for this challenge and know that it will end with you victorious—with your new energetic self overcoming weight problems and creating the life of your dreams. Remember, anything you have ever desired in your life that was huge, important, or amazing required heart, discipline and an enthusiastic presence of mind to carry it through to fruition. If you feel like you've never achieved something like this before, then let me be the first to welcome you to your potential!

> ### Exercise for Life
>
> You cannot think just one positive thought and hope it will carry you optimistically for life. Likewise, you cannot exercise just one time and hope to enjoy a lifetime of fitness. To create lifelong success with your health—to live with abundant energy, ideal weight, manageable stress, passionate relationships, and fulfilled well-being—persist daily in your commitment to fitness.

Now is the time to start achieving. See this fitness project as a working model able to adjust and change with your needs. Stick with it every day and wait with excitement to see where it takes you. I promise you, you'll love the journey. True movement will make you feel free and inspired. True movement will allow you to gain fitness without having to feel fatigued. And true movement will honor you and your personal needs and support you in being your best, without shame or pain.

Respect yourself. Start moving your body with reverence and begin believing in your commitments.

Follow through on this life plan. You can do it.

7

The NutriSystem Nourish Exercise Plan

Your Choose-to-Move Program

I developed the NutriSystem Nourish Exercise Plan to give people of all different exercise abilities and body types a simple way to fit exercise into their daily routines. Regardless of your age or ability level, the NutriSystem Nourish Exercise Plan doesn't just make exercise doable—it makes it enjoyable. The program is based on a simple premise: *choice.* While the plan outlines a basic structure, you choose the exercises to complete it.

Each level of the 4-week program—beginner, intermediate, and advanced—contains three basic elements:

1. A cardiovascular (cardio) routine
2. A resistance routine
3. A simple yoga routine

There are three different cardio routines for you to choose from. They range in length from about 10 minutes to about 25 or 30 minutes. Choosing which routine to start with is up to you.

There are also two resistance routines for you to choose from. You can perform either or both of these each week. If you have some favorite exercises, feel free to add your own or substitute yours for some of my suggestions.

The NutriSystem Nourish yoga routine is a combination of 14 yoga postures that are designed to activate your muscles, relieve tension, and produce a feeling of wellness. The yoga routine for beginners should take about 10 minutes, but you have the ability to choose to hold postures longer for an extended workout.

Exercise worksheets are also included for each element (cardio, resistance, and yoga). They provide you with the guidance you need and a sample goal based on your fitness level. You should use them like checklists to make staying on track simple. It is important that you make the effort to use these sheets to track your progress and strive to reach your goals. Feel free to photocopy the sheets out of your book, or log on to www.nutrisystem.com to print out a free version of all the NutriSystem Nourish Exercise Plan worksheets. Recording this information will help you stay focused and will make you more successful in the long run. Studies confirm that people who keep track of their diet and exercise have greater long-term success with their program, so I suggest taking some time to familiarize yourself with each routine and its worksheet before you begin. I also always recommend seeing your doctor for screening tests and advice prior to beginning any exercise program.

Rest assured that even if you have never exercised before or are returning to movement after you've been away for a while, you will find success with this program. Remember, movement is freedom. The more you move, the more fit you become and the easier it is to breathe deeply and develop muscles. The muscles that I'm talking about are not just the physical muscles attached to your skeleton but your mental, emotional, and spiritual muscles. When you flex your mental and emotional muscles, you become more self-aware and self-confident.

Regardless of how you got to this point, regardless of your weight, your size, or your level of fitness, you deserve a movement plan that supports your fitness and lifestyle goals. Here it is!

Determining Your Fitness Level

Beginning Again—First Steps

Congratulations on starting your Choose-to-Move Exercise Program. In case you're wondering, it starts today and continues for the rest of your life. As either a person just returning to exercise or someone who has been less active for a considerable length of time, your main goal is consistency. Focus on what you can do every day, not what you can't. At the beginning of your program you may not be able to walk at an increased pace for 20 minutes, but you *can* walk for 10 minutes. Every activity, every step, every yoga posture is improvement. You *can* succeed. You *will* succeed. My 4-week program for beginners is intended to help you connect with your body and reconnect to the idea of regular movement. Each workout should take you about 10 to 20 minutes. Low intensity will let you get used to exercising again. Feel free to add time to your workouts or do more than the goal of 5 during the first 2 weeks.

Week 1
Cardio	2 routines × 10 minutes
Resistance	2 routines × 10 minutes
Yoga	1 routine × 10 minutes

Week 2
Cardio	2 routines × 10 minutes
Resistance	2 routines × 10 minutes
Yoga	1 routine × 10 minutes

Week 3
Cardio	2 routines × 10 minutes
Resistance	2 routines × 10 minutes
Yoga	2 routines × 10 minutes

Week 4
Cardio	2 routines × 10 minutes
Resistance	2 routines × 10 minutes
Yoga	2 routines × 10 minutes

Intermediate Exercise—Take the Middle Ground

At the intermediate level you will be able to do some more difficult exercises and perform cardio routines that are longer in duration. At this level, focus on setting up a routine you can stick to. Track your workouts and hold yourself to them. Adding a more structured resistance and cardio program will help improve your weight loss and start to build the long, lean muscles that support increased metabolism. The 4-week intermediate routine is designed to help people who are relatively active refocus and reenergize.

Week 1
Cardio   3 routines × 15 minutes
Resistance   2 routines × 15 minutes
Yoga   2 routines × 15 minutes

Week 2
Cardio   3 routines × 15 minutes
Resistance   2 routines × 15 minutes
Yoga   2 routines × 15 minutes

Week 3
Cardio   3 routines × 15 minutes
Resistance   3 routines × 15 minutes
Yoga   2 routines × 15 minutes

Week 4
Cardio   3 routines × 15 minutes
Resistance   3 routines × 15 minutes
Yoga   2 routines × 15 minutes

Advancing Your Cause—Advanced Fitness

Starting your Choose-to-Move Exercise Program at the advanced level is a great challenge. It means you are currently exercising 2 to 4 times each week for at least 45 minutes, and consider yourself physically fit. The advanced program is a great way to support weight loss and give your metabolism a boost, while also lowering stress levels and gaining more energy. My 4-week advanced program will provide the challenge and advanced training to help the active person build strong, lean muscle.

Week 1
Cardio   4 routines × 20 minutes
Resistance   3 routines × 20 minutes
Yoga   3 routines × 15 minutes

Week 2

Cardio	4 routines × 20 minutes
Resistance	3 routines × 20 minutes
Yoga	3 routines × 15 minutes

Week 3

Cardio	4 routines × 20 minutes
Resistance	4 routines × 20 minutes
Yoga	4 routines × 15 minutes

Week 4

Cardio	4 routines × 20 minutes
Resistance	4 routines × 20 minutes
Yoga	4 routines × 15 minutes

With all of the NutriSystem Nourish Exercise Plan levels and programs, time and intensity increase gradually over the 4 weeks, but you should always feel free to return to the earlier programs if the movements become too intense too quickly. You are the best judge when it comes to your body. Listen to the signals it sends. But don't be afraid to increase your pace, resistance or number of workouts if you feel so motivated, keeping in mind that you are embarking on a lifestyle journey, not an overnight quick fix. Don't compare your progress to other people's or to how your body reacted to exercise in the past. Little advances form the groundwork for long-term success. The NutriSystem Nourish Exercise Plan is designed to give you the most amount of freedom to make movement and exercise a daily part of your life.

NutriSystem Nourish 4-week Choose-to-Move Plan Overview

B = Beginner   I = Intermediate   A = Advanced

Choose your fitness level. Add a check mark each time you perform a cardio, resistance, or yoga routine. Total your routines at the end of each week to chart your progress and measure your success.

Week 1 Level:	Day 1	Day 2	Day 3	Day 4	Day 5	Day 6	Day 7	Total	Goal B	I	A
Cardio									2	3	4
Resistance									2	2	3
Yoga									1	2	3

Week 2 Level:	Day 8	Day 9	Day 10	Day 11	Day 12	Day 13	Day 14	Total	Goal B	I	A
Cardio									2	3	4
Resistance									2	2	3
Yoga									1	2	3

Week 3 Level:	Day 15	Day 16	Day 17	Day 18	Day 19	Day 20	Day 21	Total	Goal B	I	A
Cardio									2	3	4
Resistance									2	3	4
Yoga									2	2	4

Week 4 Level:	Day 22	Day 23	Day 24	Day 25	Day 26	Day 27	Day 28	Total	Goal B	I	A
Cardio									2	3	4
Resistance									2	3	4
Yoga									2	2	4

4-Week Total					22	34	44

Free printable versions of all NutriSystem Nourish worksheets can be found at www.nutrisystem.com.

NutriSystem Nourish Cardiovascular Routines

There are three cardiovascular routines that you can choose from, and they all center around walking. During the active walk portion of your exercise program, you should be walking at a slightly rushed pace. At no point should you find yourself winded or out of breath. Walk at a pace that allows you to breathe easily and comfortably.

Each of your walking sessions should include a 5-minute warm-up and 5 to10 minutes of cooling down. Please don't ignore the benefits of a warm-up and a cool-down. I suggest always having a bottle of water with you to help you stay hydrated and a small towel to wipe away excess perspiration.

Dress the Part!

When you engage in any movement or exercise activity, wear something that breathes well. Also, you should wear clothes that you actually like because it will help you feel good while you are moving. You want to maximize comfort, but you don't want to wear clothes that are too baggy because they will end up chafing your skin. You also want to prevent skin from rubbing against skin. A pair of leggings with a sports bra and T-shirt could be a great choice for women, while men might want to choose some good-fitting sweatpants or athletic shorts and a comfortable T-shirt.

Beginner

If you are a beginner, you will focus your attention for the next 4 weeks on a mild cardiovascular exercise. Your main goal should be to get in a minimum of two 10-minute walks each week. Feel free to lengthen your walk to 15 minutes as you feel more comfortable and stronger.

Warm-Up: 5 minutes

Active Walk: 10–15 minutes*

Cool-Down: 5 minutes

Intermediate

If you are an intermediate-level exerciser, you will get a solid cardiovascular workout and will be focusing on finding a routine that you can keep. As an intermediate exerciser, it is important to take your weekly goals seriously while you incorporate movement into your everyday routine. Start with a 15-minute active walk and increase the time as you feel more physically fit.

Warm-Up: 5 minutes

Active Walk: 15–20 minutes*

Cool-Down: 5 minutes

Advanced

The advanced cardiovascular workout will provide active people with a great way to get more fit and have more energy throughout the day. Each walking routine is slightly longer, ranging from 20 to 30 minutes, but the benefits are well worth the increased time commitment.

Warm-Up: 5 minutes

Active Walk: 20–30 minutes*

Cool-Down: 5 minutes

NutriSystem Nourish Resistance Routines

Both of your NutriSystem Nourish resistance routines are designed to provide you with a simple, low-impact form of resistance training that will help you build strong, lean muscles and support an improved metabolism. To follow are descriptions of each exercise included in the routines, plus a worksheet that outlines how many reps and sets to do, depending upon your chosen level. You can buy a resistance cord at most sporting goods and fitness stores.

RESISTANCE ROUTINE A

1. Seated Twist

The movement: Sit in a chair and place your feet hip width apart. Your thighs and calves should be at a 90-degree angle (or as much as possible). Grasp the handles of your resistance cord and raise your arms to shoulder height. Extend your arms out straight in front of you and pull the cord out to the

---

*NutriSystem Nourish Exercise Note: Feel free to split up your cardio walking routines into smaller pieces if you find it easier to fit them into your day that way.

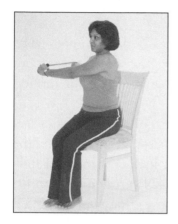

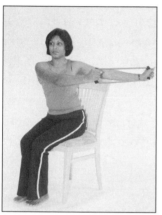

sides, working and toning your arms and shoulders and activating the circulation of blood and oxygen in your upper body. Breathe deeply, maintaining a long spine while keeping the cord stretched. Inhale and release the tension on the band. The movement should be even and smooth. Count up 2, hold, and count down 2. Exhale as you lift; inhale as you release. Repeat for the suggested number of times according to your fitness level (see worksheet on page 138).

Inhale deeply. On the exhalation, slowly turn your torso to the left. Initiate the turn from your hips and not your waist. Focus your vision on the center of the cord while maintaining outward pressure and resistance on the cord. On each exhalation, turn deeper into the twist.

NutriSystem Nourish Exercise Note: A good alternative to performing repetitions is to simply hold the stretch with the band extended for 5 to 8 long breaths, which would be equal to one set on your 4-week Exercise Tracking Worksheet.

The Technical Terms

What is a repetition or rep? A repetition or rep is performing a resistance training exercise one time. Your NutriSystem Nourish program recommends using the appropriate strength resistance band (or handheld weights) that allow you to perform anywhere from 5 to 10 repetitions of each exercise before your muscle becomes fatigued.

What is a set? A set is a given number of repetitions of any one exercise. In your NutriSystem Nourish program, one set is equal to the number of repetitions listed on your resistance worksheet.

Beginner:	5 reps = 1 set
Intermediate:	10 reps = 1 set
Advanced:	10 reps = 1 set

Depending on your fitness level, your program suggests performing anywhere from 1 to 3 sets of each exercise.

E X E R C I S E S

2. Seated Power Rowing

This exercise is great to work your abdominals, lower back, and upper back. This combination promotes good posture and a healthy spine. It also tones your arms and stretches your legs, so you have a full range of motion throughout your hips.

The movement: With your legs extended in front of you, hold your feet and knees together. Bend your legs and wrap the resistance cord around the arches of your feet. Hold one handle of the cord in each hand and fully extend your legs. Look straight ahead and sit up tall through your spine. Your arms should be fully extended in front of you so that your hands are navel height.

Engage your abs and sit up tall to support your lower back. Drop your shoulders down, engage your latissimus (lat) muscles, and pull with your arms and hands back into your abdomen. Hold, then release back to the starting position. Repeat. Concentrate on exhaling as you pull in and inhale as you release.

NutriSystem Nourish Exercise Note: During this exercise you will want to sit up tall and engage your abdomen and squeeze your buttocks to avoid leaning back and forth to gain leverage.

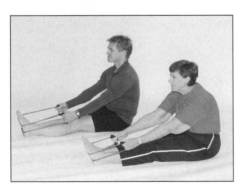 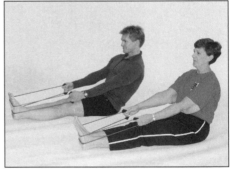

3. Side Raises

This exercise works the outsides of your shoulders. The medial deltoid is the muscle that allows you to lift your arms out to your sides. If you want to build wider, more athletic-look shoulders, this is the exercise for you.

The movement: Position yourself on your sit-bones squarely on the front edge of a chair. Place your feet about hip width apart and position your right foot in front of your left, with both feet firmly planted on the floor. Place your resistance band under the arch of your left foot. Hold the opposite handle of the band in the palm of your right hand with the cord extended across and under your right leg.

With your left hand hold the edge of the chair next to your left hip. Press down firmly with your left hand to stabilize your body during the exercise. Extend your right arm straight down alongside your right hip, keeping your spine erect, shoulders square and level. Focus on keeping your right elbow rotated out and facing backward, with the palm of your right hand facing down. Keep your elbow rotated back and feel the resistance on the outside of your shoulder. Use your buttocks and abs for more stability during the exercise.

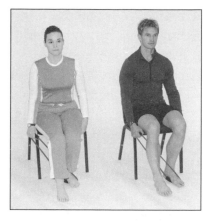

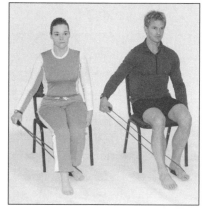

Inhale. As you exhale, engage your abs and raise your right hand straight out to the side as high as you can without forcing the movement. Hold, then release back down. With smooth movements exhale and raise up, hold, and count to 2. Then inhale as you release. Perform the suggested number of repetitions for your fitness level and repeat on the opposite side.

NutriSystem Nourish Exercise Note: To gain leverage you may tend to lean away from the movement. Spreading your feet slightly apart can help stabilize your core and improve balance. Remember to engage your buttocks and abdominal muscles for better control.

4. Standing Triceps Extensions

This exercise will help to define your triceps and also tone and strengthen your abs and legs.

The movement: Standing tall with your feet together, reach behind you with your left arm as if you were going to scratch your back. Turn your left palm so that it's facing up. Take the circle band in your right hand and reach back over your right shoulder. Grab the opposite end of the band with your left hand. Now stand tall with firm legs and your feet pressing firmly into the floor. Bring your right upper arm parallel to the floor so that your elbow is pointing forward. Keep your shoulders square and parallel to the floor. Your left arm should remain in a comfortable position. Keep in mind that your left arm and hand work to hold the band. Before you start, try pulling slightly on the band with your right hand to feel the tension.

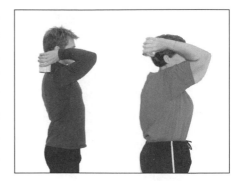

Engaging your abs, extend your right hand forward, keeping your arm at shoulder height. Squeeze your triceps muscle and slowly release. Repeat. Your upper arm should remain stable and the only movement should be your forearm moving like a lever, forward and

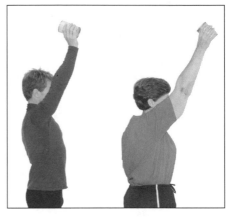

back—the contraction of your triceps. Keep the movement steady and active; don't move too slowly. Exhale as you reach and inhale as you release back. Perform the suggested number of repetitions for your fitness level. Switch arms and repeat.

NutriSystem Nourish Exercise Note: If you're a beginner and you feel unstable, spread your feet slightly apart to widen your foundation. You can also replace the resistance band with a small handheld dumbbell or 12-ounce can of soup.

5. Side-Lying Leg Raises

This exercise concentrates on toning and strengthening your hips and waist. The movement also promotes greater mobility in your hips, waist, and pelvis.

The movement: Start by lying on your left side with your legs together and fully extended. With your head resting on your hand and elbow, place your right hand directly in front of your abdomen at your navel. Your shoulder and upper arm should form a 90-degree angle. Concentrate on keeping your hips and waist level and your hipbones stacked.

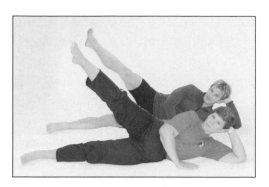

Extend your left leg while engaging your abs. Press firmly into the floor with your right hand for support and reach out with your left elbow. Press down with your upper arm as you inhale. During your exhale, raise your right leg straight up from your hip to just above your head height. Hold this for a count of 2 and release. Repeat for the number of repetitions suggested for your fitness level. Switch sides and repeat.

NutriSystem Nourish Exercise Note: Be careful not to roll your body forward and backward. Active and engaged abdominal muscles will help stabilize your body during this exercise. Keep your lower leg firm for support. Raise your leg only as far as is comfortable for you without rolling. Be careful not to overextend.

6. Ab Crunches

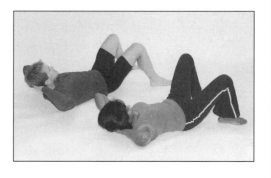

Practicing this exercise throughout the day not only helps relieve stress but also helps to calm the body and draw positive focus to your breathing. Plus toning and strengthening your abs helps to support your lower back and promote healthy posture.

The movement: Lie flat on your back with your knees bent, feet about hip width apart. With your feet a comfortable distance from your buttocks, place your hands behind your head at the base of your skull. Keep your neck long and relaxed.

Inhale. As you exhale, engage your abdomen by lifting your head and upper shoulders off the floor. This is the starting and finishing position for this exercise. Place equal pressure on the heels, balls, and toes of your feet. Concentrate on keeping your back flat on the floor and your buttocks engaged. Be sure not to use your hands to pull your head forward. Finish the movement by exhaling and engaging your upper abdominals, pulling your shoulder blades off the floor. Stop when you feel your shoulder blades rise off the floor. Hold for a count of 3 and release back to the starting position. Inhale and repeat for the number of repetitions suggested for your fitness level.

NutriSystem Nourish Exercise Note: Use your breathing to assist you in engaging your abs and reaching and lifting your shoulder blades off the floor. Don't arch your back or force leverage with your buttocks. Keep a smooth motion to avoid compressing your back or straining your neck. Maintain firm legs and a long spine and think control. For beginners who aren't strong enough to hold the lift at the starting point, I suggest starting by lying flat on your back to work your lower abs.

RESISTANCE ROUTINE B

1. Concentration Curls

We think of bicep curls as exercises that tone our arms. In addition to shapely arms, curls also help keep your elbow and wrist joints strong, which helps to prevent chronic ailments such as carpal tunnel syndrome and tendonitis.

The movement: Place your sit bones squarely on the front edge of a chair. Position your feet about hip width apart to create a strong base. Keeping your knees directly over your ankles, place your resistance band under your left foot. Hold the other end of the band between the second and third knuckles of your other hand. Extend your arm down while sitting up tall. Use your right hand on your right knee to support your torso. Keep your spine erect and your shoulders square.

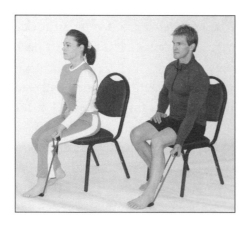
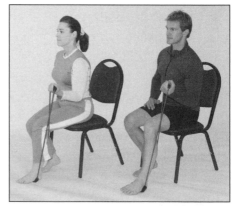

Slowly pull the circle band, focusing all your attention on the movement of your forearm and bicep. Concentrate on keeping your body steady and stable. Pull upward until your forearm is parallel to the floor, hold, squeeze your bicep, and slowly release until your arm is fully extended. Repeat for the recommended number of repetitions for your fitness level. Switch arms and repeat.

NutriSystem Nourish Exercise Note: The only motion should be your forearm swinging upward and the contraction and relaxation of your bicep muscle. Exhale as you pull and inhale as you release your bicep. Keep the movement slow and simple. Keep your body strong and hold the core of your body up tall. Press firmly through the balls and heels of your feet to gain stability.

2. Seated Overhead Back Stretch

This is a good exercise for stretching your back while toning your arms.

The movement: Hold your arms at shoulder height and grasp your resistance cord. Apply tension on the band and inhale. Raise your arms straight overhead while exhaling, reach-ing tall through your spine. Relax your shoulders while pulling firmly outward on the handles of the band.

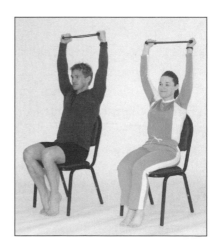

Maintain the tension in the cord for a count of 1. Inhale and lower your arms. Repeat for the number of repetitions suggested for your fitness level.

NutriSystem Nourish Exercise Note: A good alternative to performing repeti-tions is to simply hold the stretch above your head for 5 to 8 long breaths, which would be equal to one set on your 4-week Exercise Tracking Worksheet.

3. Modified Seated Forward Bend

This exercise focuses on stretching your hamstrings to create additional length in your lower spine, which helps maintain a healthy back. Perform this exercise when you feel tension building in your lower back or when you simply need to unwind.

The movement: Grasp one handle of your resistance band in each hand, inhale, and gently pull your torso downward while exhaling, resting your chest on your thighs. Breathe deeply and comfortably. If your breath is irregular, back off the stretch slightly until you can maintain an even, comfortable breathing pattern. Keep the tension on the cord to work and tone your arms while stretching your lower back, hips, and hamstrings. Hold for a count of 2, then release.

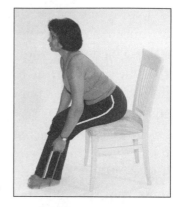

NutriSystem Nourish Exercise Note: A good alternative to performing repetitions is to simply hold the stretch with your head extended downward for 5 to 8 long breaths, which would be equal to one set on your 4-week Exercise Tracking Worksheet.

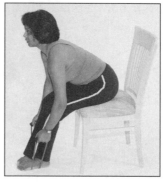

4. Front Raises

This exercise helps to strengthen your shoulder joints and enhance shoulder mobility by strengthening smaller muscles that may be inactive.

The movement: Position yourself on your sit bones squarely on the front edge of a chair. Place your feet about hip width apart and align your knees directly over your ankles. Place your resistance band under the arch of your right foot. Hold the other handle of the band in the palm of your right hand. With your left hand, grip the edge of the chair next to your left hip. Pressing down firmly with your left hand will help stabilize your body during the exercise. Extend your right arm straight out directly above your right knee, keeping your spine erect with your shoulders square and level. Keep your right elbow facing out to your side and the palm of your right hand facing down at all times. This means rotating your arm to the outside; you will feel this when you begin the movement. Work to keep your elbow rotated outward and focus all resistance on your shoulder. Press firmly through your feet and activate your legs. Concentrate on engaging your abs and buttocks. Perform as many repetitions as recommended for your fitness level, switch hands, and repeat.

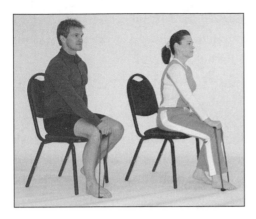 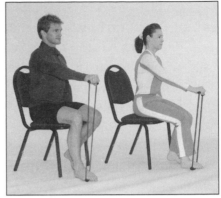

Inhale. As you exhale, engage your abs and raise your right hand straight up to shoulder height, hold, and release back down to your knee. Repeat. The movement should be even and smooth. Count up 2, hold, and count down 2. Exhale as you lift and inhale as you release.

NutriSystem Nourish Exercise Note: Try not to lean forward or backward. To prevent this, spread your feet slightly until you have stabilized the core of your body and found your balance.

5. Focus Rowing

This exercise allows you to fully concentrate on the movement of one arm at a time.

The movement: Sit upright with your legs extended 3 to 4 feet apart. Place the resistance cord around your right foot and grasp the other end of the cord with both hands. Press through your heels and keep your legs firm, being careful not to lock your knees. Maintain a stable yet comfortable

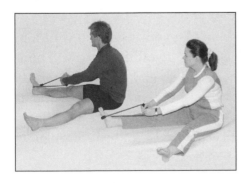 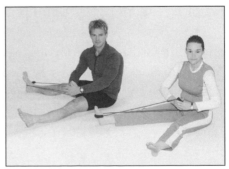

E X E R C I S E S

position that allows your shoulders to stay square and level with your waist and the floor. Engage your abs and fully extend your arms toward your right foot. Keep your hands at navel height. Exhale and pull your arms directly back alongside your rib cage. Hold and release. Do the number of repetitions suggested for your fitness level.

NutriSystem Nourish Exercise Note: To prevent leaning backward and forward, sit up tall and engage your abdominals to support your torso. Push firmly with your supporting hand, keeping your arm firm and stable. For more control, follow the movement of your arm with your eyes. Exhale as you pull and inhale as you release.

6. Leg Raise Ab Crunch

I call this exercise the concentration curl of abdominal work because it requires total focus on the abdominal muscles to get the maximum benefit. This exercise can give you a firm, flat stomach, and helps to support a healthy lower back and spine.

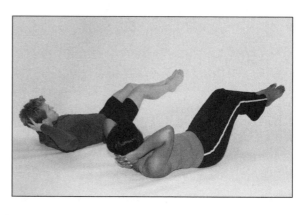

The movement: Lie flat on your back with your feet together and heels touching. Stretch your body long and place your hands behind your head for support.

Inhale. As you exhale, activate your lower abdominal wall and lift your feet 6 to 8 inches off the floor. You should engage your entire abdominal wall for a count of 3, and then release slowly back to the floor. Do the number of repetitions suggested for your fitness level.

NutriSystem Nourish Exercise Note: Don't lift your legs from your hips and waist; instead, use your abs to pull your legs up off the floor with minimal help from your hips. Keep your neck and shoulders relaxed and try not to arch your back. Press firmly down with your hands to help support your legs and release tension from your lower back. If you're a beginner, start with your knees slightly bent and keep your knees bent throughout the exercise.

Your NutriSystem Nourish Resistance Worksheets

Following are exercise worksheets that provide you with the basic structure of your exercise plan in an easy-to-follow format. Once you choose a fitness level—beginner, intermediate, or advanced—refer to the worksheet to see what your goals are for each week. For each week, I suggest a certain number of workouts for each exercise.

If it is easier, I encourage you to split up your exercises into smaller workouts throughout the day. You don't always have to devote large blocks of time to receive the health and weight-loss benefits of exercise, but you should set goals and take them seriously.

Upping the Intensity

Increasing your resistance. When you are ready to increase the intensity of your weight workout, first try increasing the number of repetitions of each exercise with the same amount of weight. Resistance bands come in varying amounts of resistance, so it would be useful to have several bands of different resistances. When you can comfortably do the suggested repetitions, go ahead and increase the amount of weight you are lifting by no more than one increment. For example, if you are lifting 2-pound dumbbells in each hand, go up to a 3-pound dumbbell for each hand. You should sense effort and maybe even a little discomfort, but you should never sense pain. You should always be able to breathe and speak comfortably while exercising.

Increasing your cardio. When you are ready to increase your level of fitness, try walking a little farther or bike or swim longer than you did before, and slowly increase the rate or pace of your exercise as the days and weeks pass.

Each day, after you perform either a cardio, resistance, or yoga routine, record it on your tracking sheet. If you're splitting your routine up over the course of the day, feel free to record the amount of exercise or the time you exercised in the boxes to help you keep track. This is your working tool. At the end of each week, count up the number of each of the routines and see your progress. Use your first week as a benchmark to track your advancement. If you reached the goal, wonderful. If not, don't feel bad or even discouraged. Look at how many exercises you *did* do. Each day is progress.

Free printable versions of all NutriSystem Nourish worksheet can be found at www.nutrisystem.com.

NutriSystem Nourish Resistance A—Program Worksheet

Choose your appropriate fitness level. Make sure to record your sets, repetitions, and how much resistance (what band or how much weight) for each exercise.

Choose Appropriate Level	Beginner	Intermediate	Advanced	
	Sets/Repetitions	Sets/Repetitions	Sets/Repetitions	
Goal	1 / 5	1–2 / 10	2–3 / 10	
1. Seated Twist	/	/	/	
_____ (lb.)	/	/	/	
	/	/	/	

Choose Appropriate Level	Beginner	Intermediate	Advanced	
	Sets/Repetitions	Sets/Repetitions	Sets/Repetitions	
Goal	1 / 5	1–2 / 10	2–3 / 10	
2. Seated Power Rowing	/	/	/	
_____ (lb.)	/	/	/	
	/	/	/	

Choose Appropriate Level	Beginner	Intermediate	Advanced	
	Sets/Repetitions	Sets/Repetitions	Sets/Repetitions	
Goal	1 / 5	1–2 / 10	2–3 / 10	
3. Side Raises	/	/	/	
_____ (lb.)	/	/	/	
	/	/	/	

Choose Appropriate Level	Beginner	Intermediate	Advanced
	Sets/Repetitions	Sets/Repetitions	Sets/Repetitions
Goal	1 / 5	1–2 / 10	2–3 / 10
4. Standing Triceps Extensions	/	/	/
	/	/	/
_____ (lb.)	/	/	/

Choose Appropriate Level	Beginner	Intermediate	Advanced
	Sets/Repetitions	Sets/Repetitions	Sets/Repetitions
Goal	1 / 5	1–2 / 10	2–3 / 10
5. Side-Lying Leg Raises	/	/	/
_____ (lb.)	/	/	/
	/	/	/

Choose Appropriate Level	Beginner	Intermediate	Advanced
	Sets/Repetitions	Sets/Repetitions	Sets/Repetitions
Goal	1 / 5	1–2 / 10	2–3 / 10
6. Ab Crunches	/	/	/
_____ (lb.)	/	/	/
	/	/	/

NutriSystem Nourish Resistance B—Program Worksheet

Choose your appropriate fitness level. Make sure to record your sets, repetitions, and how much resistance (what band or how much weight) below each exercise.

Choose Appropriate Level	Beginner	Intermediate	Advanced
	Sets/Repetitions	Sets/Repetitions	Sets/Repetitions
Goal	1 / 5	1–2 / 10	2–3 / 10
1. Concentration Curls	/	/	/
_____ (lb.)	/	/	/
	/	/	/

EXERCISES

Choose Appropriate Level	Beginner	Intermediate	Advanced
	Sets/Repetitions	Sets/Repetitions	Sets/Repetitions
Goal	1 / 5	1–2 / 10	2–3 / 10
2. Seated Overhead Back Stretch	/	/	/
	/	/	/
_____ (lb.)	/	/	/

Choose Appropriate Level	Beginner	Intermediate	Advanced
	Sets/Repetitions	Sets/Repetitions	Sets/Repetitions
Goal	1 / 5	1–2 / 10	2–3 / 10
3. Modified Seated Forward Bend	/	/	/
	/	/	/
_____ (lb.)	/	/	/

Choose Appropriate Level	Beginner	Intermediate	Advanced
	Sets/Repetitions	Sets/Repetitions	Sets/Repetitions
Goal	1 / 5	1–2 / 10	2–3 / 10
4. Front Raises	/	/	/
_____ (lb.)	/	/	/
	/	/	/

Choose Appropriate Level	Beginner	Intermediate	Advanced
	Sets/Repetitions	Sets/Repetitions	Sets/Repetitions
Goal	1 / 5	1–2 / 10	2–3 / 10
5. Focus Rowing	/	/	/
_____ (lb.)	/	/	/
	/	/	/

Choose Appropriate Level	Beginner	Intermediate	Advanced
	Sets/Repetitions	Sets/Repetitions	Sets/Repetitions
Goal	1 / 5	1–2 / 10	2–3 / 10
6. Leg Raise Ab Crunch	/	/	/
_____ (lb.)	/	/	/
	/	/	/

NutriSystem Nourish Yoga Routine

Your NutriSystem Nourish Yoga Routine was designed to include 14 basic yoga postures. Practicing these postures in one routine or performing them individually throughout the day is a good way to alleviate stress from your life and help your muscles to feel reenergized.

1. Standing Pose

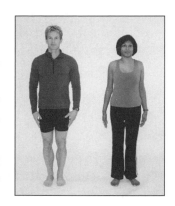

The benefit: We will begin the NutriSystem Nourish yoga routine with the standing pose. The upright and firm posture required in the standing pose reduces stress and can increase your focus.

The posture: Stand tall with your feet together. The heels and big toes of both of your feet should be touching each other. Concentrate on spreading your toes out. Extend your arms down your sides, with your fingers stretching toward the floor. Feel your body lengthen as you reach up tall through your head. Look straight ahead as you breathe deeply and consistently.

To feel the posture and find the proper position, make sure to stand with firm legs. Tighten your knees slightly and firm your buttocks. While keeping your stomach strong, lift up with your chest and spine. Keep your neck straight up, as if a rope were pulling you skyward through the center of your body. Hold this posture for 5 long, even breaths. As you gain more confidence and strength, strive to hold this pose for a full minute.

NutriSystem Nourish Exercise Note: It is helpful to balance your weight evenly between your heels and your toes. Beginners should feel free to start with their feet spread slightly apart or with their heels and back pressed firmly against a wall.

2. Standing Pose with Arms Overhead

The benefit: The standing pose with arms overhead is a great stretch and stress reliever for anyone who spends too much time sitting down. This posture helps strengthen the joints of the shoulders, arms, and wrists.

The posture: Inhale, then exhale while raising your arms upward. Your hands should remain shoulder width apart and your fingers should reach skyward. Relax your shoulders and reach as tall as you can. Hold this posture for 5 long, even breaths, working up to holding the pose for a full minute as your body becomes stronger.

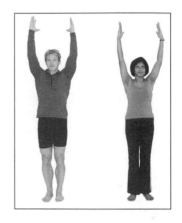

NutriSystem Nourish Exercise Note: Don't scrunch your shoulders together to reach higher. Instead, try to relax your neck and feel your shoulders fall back and down. If you're a beginner, try this pose against the wall to start.

3. Standing Forward Bend

The benefit: You'll focus on stretching and lengthening your hamstrings. You will also benefit from the calming effects that forward bending can offer your body and mind. This exercise helps to calm your nervous system and slow your heart rate while it deeply stretches and rejuvenates your spine. Perform this exercise anytime you feel the need to unwind and feel more balanced.

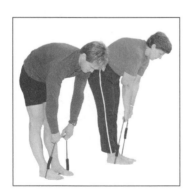

The posture: Move into the standing forward bend on the exhalation from the standing pose with arms overhead. As you exhale slowly, fold forward from your hips, keeping your knees slightly bent, and reach your hands to the floor. Feel free to place an exercise cord beneath your feet and grasp the handles to help with the stretch. Focus your vision ahead of you as you slowly begin to straighten your legs on each exhalation. Breathe deeply, concentrating on a long exhalation. Be aware that your shoulders should be relaxed and your neck flexible. Take advantage of using the cord to help you stretch and lengthen your hamstrings, but do not force the stretch by pulling your torso down with the cord. Use your breath to deepen the stretch and the cord to support you.

As your flexibility increases, work to increase the stretch by straightening your legs completely. Always keep your shoulders and neck relaxed as you reach long through your spine, extending forward from your hips.

Remove excess length in the cord by bringing your hands together and clasping both handles together. Maintain a comfortable breathing pattern and concentrate on lengthening through your spine and out of your hips. Don't force yourself forward and keep your back straight at all times. Inhale and reach with your chest. Exhale and lengthen your hamstrings up through your spine. Perform this exercise for 5 to 8 long, deep breaths, maintaining tension on the cord and deepening the stretch through your hips and lower back each time you exhale.

4. Half Up Dog and Back Stretch

The benefit: This pose is great to stretch out after performing abdominal or back exercises. This movement also helps tone your abs and is an excellent stretch for anyone who spends a lot of time standing or sitting.

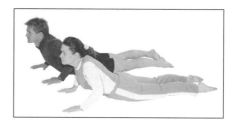

The posture: Lie face down on your stomach and place your feet hip width apart. Stretch your body out and position your hands alongside your chest, fingers pointing forward. Inhale. On the exhalation, slowly press up through your hands so that your chest lifts off the floor and you reach out through your head. Focus your vision straight ahead, reach back, and extend through your feet, always keeping your legs active. Feel the stretch in your abs and feel the tension of your lower back releasing, allowing your body to reach and lift through your chest. Breathe. Hold for a count of 3, exhale, and release. Beginners should work up to 6 repetitions, holding for 3 to 5 counts then work up to 10 repetitions, holding for 5 to 8 counts each.

NutriSystem Nourish Exercise Note: Concentrate on keeping your neck and shoulders relaxed throughout the pose. Don't overextend and compress your lower back. Maintain active legs and stretch out long through your feet. You should be able to comfortably breathe while holding your chest in the raised position.

5. Staff Pose

The benefit: Consistently practicing the staff pose, particularly if you sit for long periods of time during the day, will help to correct your posture, alleviate tension in your spine and legs, and stimulate your abdomen and pelvic regions for better circulation.

The posture: Extend your legs out in front of you with your feet side by

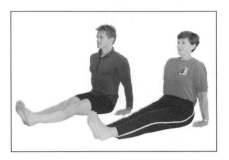

side and touching each other. Position yourself by pulling the flesh of your buttocks back so that you are seated on your sit-bones. Place both hands on the floor directly alongside your hips, fingers pointing forward. Relax and release your shoulder blades down and from your ears as you reach tall through your spine. Relax your abdomen and feel the tension release as you take long, deep breaths. Press your hands down to lift your spine and make sure to keep your shoulders and abdomen relaxed. Extend long through your heels and activate your legs to create length through your hamstrings. Breathe. Hold this posture for 5 long, even breaths to start and work toward a goal of holding the pose for a full minute.

If you're a beginner or you're not very flexible in your hips and waist, perform this posture sitting with a yoga brick positioned directly under your sit-bones.

NutriSystem Nourish Exercise Note: Find balance in your posture. Lift straight up and be careful not to lean to one side or the other. Focus on keeping your shoulders and waist level, not leaning forward or backward. Press firmly through your hands for support. Yoga bricks, mats, straps and other accessories can be purchased at most sporting goods stores.

6. Kneeling Pose

The benefit: This posture is recommended if you stand or sit for long periods of time and can relieve stiffness in your hips and knees. The kneeling pose can also reduce inflammation in your legs, and it alleviates pain in your feet, ankles, and calves. It also helps increase blood circulation throughout your body.

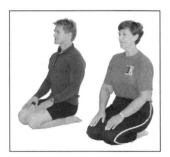

The posture: Let yourself crouch in a kneeling position with your knees about hip width apart and your buttocks resting comfortably between your feet and ankles. If possible, try to rest your buttocks to the floor. Inhale to start. As you exhale, interlace your fingers, turning your palms inside out as you raise your arms overhead.

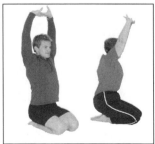

Relax your legs and hips and concentrate on reaching long through your spine. On each exhalation, release your shoulder blades down and away from your neck, keeping your neck flexible. Keep your torso balanced evenly over your hips and waist. Focus on good posture and try not to lean forward or backward. Hold this posture for 5 long, even breaths with the goal of eventually holding the pose for a full minute as you become stronger.

NutriSystem Nourish Exercise Note: If your legs are not very flexible, use a blanket to raise your hips off the floor so that you can comfortably sit and hold this position.

7. Kneeling Pose with Twist

The benefit: Here you'll increase the benefits of the kneeling pose by adding a simple twisting motion. The twist helps relieve pressure in your lower back and relaxes the muscles in your abdomen, aiding in overall body circulation and digestion. This posture also helps to expand your chest and to increase your breathing capacity.

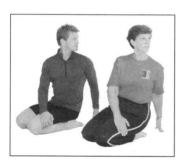

The posture: From the kneeling pose release your arms down to the floor alongside your hips. Inhale deeply. As you exhale, slowly twist your upper body to the left. Place your left hand on the floor behind your left hip. Place your right hand on your left thigh just above your knee. On each exhalation, try to increase the twist and concentrate on lifting through your spine. Make sure to turn your shoulders and spine from the waist. Turn your head into the twist as you exhale. Hold and twist with each exhalation for 3 to 5 deep breaths. Release slowly and repeat on the other side.

NutriSystem Nourish Exercise Note: If you're not flexible through your shoulders, spine, and hips, place a yoga brick directly behind your hip for added support.

8. Seated Forward Bend

The benefit: The seated forward bend calms your nervous system and alleviates stress and tension. The posture stretches the entire back of your body from your head to your feet. It will also help your leg muscles become more flexible, which can help to support your lower back.

The posture: From the kneeling pose, inhale deeply. As you exhale, reach tall through your spine and bend forward from your waist, reaching your hands toward your feet. Relax your neck and shoulders and lift through your chest. Breathe deeply and comfortably. On each exhalation,

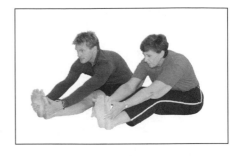

relax deeper into the stretch. Bend farther forward as you bring your chest closer to your thighs. To begin, hold this posture for 5 long, even breaths as you work toward a goal of holding this pose for a full minute.

NutriSystem Nourish Exercise Note: If you are a beginner or if your hamstrings are less flexible, a yoga strap can be used to help extend your arms so that you can comfortably bend forward from your hips. If you find that you're reaching with your head and creating a curve in your back, release the pose and use a strap until you gain more flexibility. Beginners can also use a yoga brick under their bottoms for added height in the hips so that they can perform the pose more comfortably.

9. Wide-Leg Seated Forward Bend

The benefit: This exercise promotes a deep opening of your hips and hamstrings, relieving tension in your lower back and sacrum. The wide-leg position helps stimulate your abdomen to relieve tension.

The posture: From the seated forward bend, spread your legs as far apart as possible without leaning backward. With your hands next to your hips, press down. As you inhale, lift your chest. As you exhale, slowly lean forward from your hips, keeping your back straight while

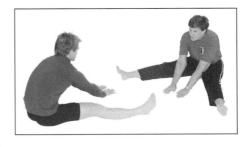

placing your hands on the floor in front of you. Hold the stretch at arm length, concentrating on extending through your spine. Make sure to keep your legs active as you reach out firmly through your heels. Focus on pressing the backs of your knees to the floor. Breathe deeply and concentrate, reaching up through your spine and lifting your chest. As you get comfortable in the stretch, lean farther forward. Keep your neck and shoulders relaxed. Hold this stretch for 5 to 8 long, even breaths.

NutriSystem Nourish Exercise Note: If you're a beginner or have hips and hamstrings that are less flexible, start with your knees slightly bent and work up to stretching with straight legs.

10. Bridge

The benefit: The bridge pose helps tone your quads, hamstrings, and abs while tightening your buttock muscles. This exercise also helps stabilize your hips and waist. Including this exercise in your routine after performing abdominal exercises helps to stretch the abs.

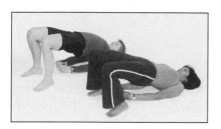

The posture: Lie flat on your back with your feet about hip width apart. Stretch your body long and reach up through the top of your head. Place your hands next to your buttocks for support.

Bend your knees so that your feet are flat on the floor. Move your hands out slightly wider than shoulder width and inhale. As you exhale, squeeze your buttock muscles together and press your pelvic bone to the sky. Reach strong through your waist and elevate your hips to the bridge position. Breathe. Hold for a count of 3, then exhale and release. Beginners should start with 6 repetitions for 3 to 5 counts and work toward 10 repetitions, holding for 5 to 8 counts as muscles get stronger.

NutriSystem Nourish Exercise Note: Keep your neck relaxed and look straight up. Be careful not to overextend and compress your chest into your neck. Maintain active legs and press your feet firmly into the floor. Use your arms for balance and support and raise your hips only as far as is comfortable for you.

11. Reclined Single-Leg Twist

The benefit: This exercise promotes a deep stretch in your lower back and waist. It's excellent for correcting an uneven posture and great for those who sit or stand for long periods each day. It is also a good stretch to promote a healthy lower back. Feel free to perform it throughout the day to alleviate stress and lower back tension.

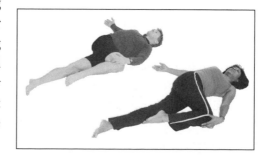

The posture: Sitting with your legs extended out in front of you, slowly lower your torso to the floor, extending up through your spine and down through your heels. Bend your right leg and bring your right knee leftward to a 90-degree angle across your body. Hold your right knee with your left hand and extend your right arm out to the side at shoulder height above you. Inhale and lengthen up through your spine and down through the bottom of your left foot. Exhale. Rotate your chest to the right and gently push your right knee to the floor. Keep your left leg extended and activated. Allow your left leg to naturally rotate to the left as you deepen the stretch. Breathe deeply. Hold this stretch for 5 to 8 long, even breaths. Release and perform on the other side.

12. Child's Pose

The benefit: The child's pose allows you to relieve pressure on your lower back and realign your spine. Resting your forehead on your forearms helps to relieve tension in your head. This posture also helps you develop good abdominal breathing.

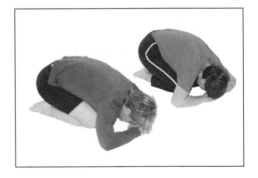

The posture: Start in a kneeling position with your buttocks on your heels. Sit tall and inhale deeply. As you exhale, slowly drop your torso forward. Rest your chest and abdomen on your thighs. Fold your arms in front of you and rest your forehead on your forearms. Allow your entire upper body to rest comfortably. Let your legs relax and spread open slightly, if necessary. You should feel tension release from your back and your body weight should begin to rest on your thighs. Take 5 long, even breaths at the start and work up to holding the pose for a full minute as you gain confidence and strength.

13. Supported Relaxation Pose

The benefit: In the supported relaxation pose, you'll use a yoga brick or rolled yoga mat to elevate your chest and diaphragm. This will increase your breathing capacity and stimulate the flow of oxygen throughout your body. This posture is not meant to be meditative but should stimulate energy flow to help reduce stress.

The posture: Sit with your legs extended in front of you. Slowly roll onto your right side. Use your arms to press yourself up to a seated position and place the end of a bolster against your lower back and hips. Slowly release

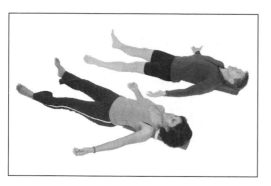

yourself down onto the bolster with your spine and head resting on the top. You should feel a lift through your chest and a stretch through your abdomen. With your hips and waist raised slightly off the floor, allow your shoulders to open out to the sides and your arms to rest comfortably out and away from your body, palms facing upward. Move your feet about shoulder width apart and let your legs naturally fall open from your hips. Feel your entire body sink into the floor and bolster. Breathe deeply and comfortably while concentrating on relaxing your body from head to toe. Hold this posture for up to 3 minutes.

14. Relaxation Pose

The benefit: In the relaxation pose you are practicing the art of remaining motionless. This will help you keep your mind still, bringing you into a state of conscious relaxation. You will feel the stress release and all the muscles in your body relax. The practice of conscious relaxation invigorates your body and refreshes your mind.

The posture: From the supported relaxation pose, slowly roll onto your right side and take five long, deep breaths to awaken your mind. Use your arms to press yourself up to a seated position while keeping your legs extended. Remove the yoga brick or mat and slowly lower yourself back

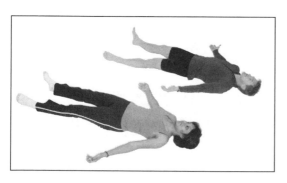

down to the floor. Position your feet just wider than shoulder width apart, allowing your legs to naturally fall open from your hips. Relax your neck and release your shoulders down. Let your arms rest slightly out and away from your sides, palms facing upward. Breathe deeply and evenly; close your eyes and feel your body sink into the floor. Stay in this pose for up to 15 minutes. Concentrate on deep breaths with long, slow exhalations. Feel your body relax and the tension release.

To come out of the pose, slowly roll onto your right side and take a few long, deep breaths to awaken your mind. Use your arms to press yourself up to a seated position and cross your legs in front of you. Rest in the seated cross-legged position for a few moments.

NutriSystem Nourish Yoga Worksheet

Use this sheet as an easy reference guide when you are performing your yoga routine. Feel free to lengthen or shorten your yoga routine as time allows. The yoga postures can be performed in one long routine or as separate moves throughout the day to help you feel energized and alleviate stress.

Pose	Breathing	Hints	
1. Standing Pose	Breathe deeply and consistently.	Keep your stomach strong and lift your chest, spine, and neck upward as if being pulled by a rope.	
2. Standing Pose with Arms Overhead	Inhale and exhale for 5 long, even breaths.	Keep your hands shoulder width apart with fingers reaching skyward.	
3. Standing Forward Bend	Inhale through your spine and exhale slowly as you fold forward. Hold for 5 to 8 long, deep breaths.	Make sure to keep your neck and shoulders relaxed as you use the cord to help lengthen your hamstrings.	
4. Half Up Dog and Back Stretch	Inhale deeply, then exhale while pressing through your hands.	Stretch your body long and feel the tension release in your abs and lower back. Focus your vision straight ahead.	
5. Staff Pose	At the start, hold this posture for 5 long, even breaths, working up to holding the pose for 1 minute.	Relax your shoulder blades and release the tension in your abdomen. Extend through your heels and activate your legs.	

Pose	Breathing	Hints	
6. Kneeling Pose	At the start, hold this posture for 5 even, long breaths, working up to holding the pose for 1 minute.	Concentrate on keeping your torso balanced over your hips by reaching tall through your arms	
7. Kneeling Pose with Twist	Hold the twist for 3 to 5 deep, even breaths.	Place your right hand on your left thigh and increase your twist on each exhalation.	
8. Seated Forward Bend	At the start, hold this posture for 5 even, long breaths, working up to holding the pose for 1 minute.	Relax your neck and shoulders and lift through your chest. Bend farther on each exhalation.	
9. Wide-Leg Seated Forward Bend	Lift your chest as you inhale and bend forward as you exhale. Hold this pose for 5 to 8 long, even breaths.	Concentrate on keeping your back straight and pressing the backs of your knees to the floor.	
10. Bridge	Inhale and hold for a count of 1 before exhaling. Hold the pose for a count of 3, working up to a count of 8 as you get stronger.	Have your hands just past shoulder width apart and concentrate and try to keep your neck relaxed, legs firm, and feet firmly pressed into the floor.	
11. Reclined Single-Leg Twist.	Lift your chest as you inhale and bend forward as you exhale. Hold this pose for 5 to 8 long, even breaths.	Lengthen through your spine and the bottom of your foot. Gently push your right knee to the floor.	
12. Child's Pose	At the start, hold this posture for 5 even, long breaths, working up to holding the pose for 1 minute.	With your forehead resting on your arms, allow your upper body to rest comfortably on your thighs, releasing tension from your back.	
13. Supported Relaxation Pose	Elevate chest and hold this pose for up to 3 minutes, breathing deeply and comfortably.	Allow your shoulders to open out to your side and keep your arms relaxed with your palms facing upward.	
14. Relaxation Pose	Stay in this pose for up to 15 minutes, inhaling deeply and exhaling long, slow breaths.	With your eyes closed, concentrate on your breathing and feel your body sink into the floor.	

Free printable versions of all NutriSystem Nourish worksheets can be found at www.nutrisystem.com.

Bookend Routines

I explain the notion of these Bookend Routines in Chapter 4. They're a great way to start and end your day.

Morning Bookend Routine

Here is an example of a nice morning movement ritual.

- Begin standing with your weight balanced over your feet, arms to the side, your shoulders down and back and your gaze directed forward. Inhale and raise your arms out to your side. Exhale and bring your palms together in front of your heart.

- Inhale again and raise your hands over your head until your palms face one another. Exhale and allow your body to fold forward slowly from the hips. Depending on your flexibility, you can either place your hands on your knees, on a book by your feet or on a yoga block or down to the sides of your feet. Breathe for 5 full slow breaths. Release your hands and slowly come up, keeping your back long and straight, your arms stretched out overhead, and return to your beginning position. Repeat this forward flexing once more.

- Once you fold forward and establish your own balance, step back with your right foot so that you are in a lunge position. Maintain this position for 2 breaths, then bring your arms to your knee. Beginners should stay here.

- If you feel balanced and ready to proceed, lift your arms up over your head, balancing your weight between your legs and lengthening through your rib cage. Gaze upward and breathe for 3 full breaths. Then return to the lunge for 1 breath, step your foot back to forward bend position, and slowly come up to standing once again. Repeat on the other side.

- When you are back in the neutral standing position, jump your feet into an A stance where they are about 3 feet apart. Put your hands on your hips and lengthen your spine. Again bend forward from your hips and place your hands either on the floor or on a book or yoga brick. Breathe for 5 full breaths and come back up with an elongated spine.

- From here, hug yourself, grasping both elbows if you can.

- Next, clasp your hands behind your buttocks and squeeze your shoulder blades together. Hold this position for 5 full breaths, then extend your grasped hands out until you feel a moderate stretch in your chest and shoulder blades. Hold for 3 to 5 breaths and return to a neutral standing position.

- Bring one arm across your chest and hug it with your other arm to hold the stretch. Repeat on the other side.

- Give yourself time every morning upon waking to relax and meditate with a cup of tea, go for a walk, stretch, or get some other form of exercise.

Evening Bookend Routine

Perform 15 minutes of quiet floor exercises. Here is one example that I think you'll find wonderfully relaxing:

- Begin in a simple cross-legged seated position. Stretch your arms behind you with your fingertips on the floor turned away from your body. Inhale and lift your chest. Breathe here for 5 long breaths.

- On your last exhalation, bring your arms back toward the front of your body and walk your hands out in front of you until you feel a gentle stretch in your hips. Stay here and breathe again for another 5 seconds.

- When and if you feel ready, walk your hands out even farther until you feel an additional stretch in your back. Breathe.

- Walk your hands back up to a neutral position. From here go back into the seated position and again bring your arms behind your body and fingertips on the ground facing away from your body. Inhale and lift your chest. Exhale and allow your body to twist to the left.

- From this place of rotation, allow your right hand to come around and rest on your left knee. Inhale to lengthen your spine and exhale to further assist your twist. Breathe slowly for 5 breaths and repeat this twist on the other side.

- Return to your simple crossed-leg seated position and straighten one leg at a time out in front of you so that you are in what is called a staff pose. You may choose to sit on a blanket for additional support (this will help keep your pelvis straight). Use a yoga strap if needed to wrap around your feet. With your back straight and your shoulders down, stretch toward your shins.

- If you have greater flexibility, remove the strap and reach for your toes with your hands. Fold forward from your hips, moving toward your shins. Hold and breathe for 5 breaths. Inhale as you come up.

- Slowly roll to your side and lower yourself down to the ground so that you are resting on the floor with your legs bent. Lie on your back and pull your knees into your chest. Slowly roll left and right and feel the release in your back.

- Then allow your knees to fall to the right side and slowly turn your head and rib cage away from your bent knees to the left. Breathe for 5 slow breaths. On the last exhalation, bring your knees back into your chest and repeat the exercise on the other side.

- When you are done, come to all fours with your hands under your shoulders and knees under your hips. Press back into the child's pose, allowing your hips to move back toward your heels. Rest here as long as you'd like.

- Give yourself time every night before going to bed where you refrain from stressful conversations and stimulation, especially television and the news, and just enjoy some candlelight, a good book, or some calming music. This is a good time to dim the lights.

PART FOUR

Nourishing Success

8

Steps to Success

Resolve to Evolve

Resolve to evolve.

I love the sound of that. Weight loss and evolution really go hand in hand.

When you choose to participate in any weight-loss program, you really are saying that you'd like to evolve. The problem is that with most diets you never really do. While your resolve may surely get tested, you never really have the tools to make success happen. You quit, you fail, or you're less than pleased with your results—a far cry from having evolved to a place where you can really manage your weight.

This program is different. With the NutriSystem Nourish program, you have the means to succeed. And by resolving to do so, you actually *will* evolve! You'll actually notice things about yourself that you may have never known before, and you'll discover your strength and beauty long forgotten. You'll become the person you were meant to be.

> I have struggled with my body image most of my life. As a kid I was definitely fit, but I never felt fully comfortable in my body and I always struggled with the size of my legs and bottom. As I moved into adulthood and motherhood, it is hard to believe that I was still struggling with these same issues. I realized that the common denominator in all of my years was eating the same type of diet throughout my life. I had added more vegetables and less candy to my regimen, but I still relied heavily on starchy carbohydrates to get

me through the day. Through journaling, yoga, and choosing lower-glycemic carbohydrates, coupled with my natural love for movement, my body is finally in a place where I can happily say I am where I want to be.—Kathy, age 35

Five Steps to NutriSystem Nourish

We've discussed a lot in this book, and now you know that this program really comes down to five steps that form the foundation for your success. When you do these things, your program will come together in your own life and you'll lose weight. Here are the five things you need to do.

1. Plan to Succeed

Take the time to think about the role that food, exercise, and nourishing yourself will have in the days to come. Remember, if you take the time to plan to succeed on your weight-loss program, then you will!

- Build time into your wake-up and bedtime routines for soothing exercises that will serve as your bookends for the day. Coming into and exiting the day peacefully will increase your motivation on the NutriSystem Nourish program. Take the time to choose activities that are right for you. Deep breathing? Meditation? Yoga? Soft music? Soothing herbal tea?
- Create and respect a to-you list that puts yourself at the top of the to-do list each day.

2. Map Out Meals

Take the time to plan your menu for the day and get excited about it. You are going to be eating all day long, losing weight, and not feeling hungry.

- If you are going to cook, make sure you make time to shop for all of the ingredients you'll need.
- If you'll be enjoying NutriSystem Nourish prepared foods, select the foods you'll be eating.
- If you will be eating meals away from home, make sure that you carefully pack the foods you'll want to have with you.
- Plan out the times when you'd like to eat your five meals and snacks (approximately 3 hours apart); take your supplements and drink water.

- Remember that you control your metabolism. If you feed your body low-glycemic-index foods at regular intervals, it will respond by burning fat.

3. Think Positively

Ask yourself several times a day if you are thinking positively. Mealtimes may be a good time to check in. Remember that you can use positive thoughts as nourishment for your entire body. Thinking more positively on the inside can really help you become who you want to be on the outside.

- If you find that you have thoughts that may be discouraging your goals, pull out your mental floss by writing them down and replacing them with new, affirming thoughts. Take note of any excuses in your life, too, and practice But Reduction often!
- Add positivity props to your life whenever you can, surrounding yourself with people, objects, and experiences that aid and encourage positive change.

4. Stress Less

Remember that stress is fattening. When you are chronically stressed, you burn fewer calories, lose muscle, and tend to experience an increase in appetite. The name of the game is to decrease stress as much as possible every day.

- Incorporate deep breathing, yoga and mediation into your life and bookend routines.
- Squeeze in at least one nourishing moment every day. Whether it's a 1-minute temple massage, or a 30-minute date with a bubble bath, any time spent taking care of yourself will contribute to your self-esteem and your level of motivation in your weight-loss program.

5. Keep Moving

Create a realistic exercise program for each day that takes all of the other responsibilities in your life into consideration. Just remember that the more you exercise the faster you will lose weight.

- Start slowly and build up to a program that is right for you. Whether you're a beginner, intermediate, or advanced exerciser, choose a NutriSystem Nourish exercise plan that works for you.

- Use a combination of different movements to get the best return from your investment.
- Exercise whenever you can fit it into your schedule, but keep in mind that morning exercise jumpstarts your metabolism and keeps it elevated for hours—sometimes up to 24 hours.
- Use Metabolic Minutes to supplement your program. Whether it's the bicep curl with a soup can in the kitchen while waiting for the microwave buzzer or taking a lap around your house before you walk in the front door, it's surprising how many opportunities you can find in a day to exercise if you are looking for them.
- Use exercise as an opportunity to lift your spirit, support your weight-loss effort, and optimize your health.

By incorporating these elements into your life, you can thrive on the NutriSystem Nourish program—you'll lose weight and reshape your entire life experience.

Support When You Need It

The notion of losing weight and nourishing your life on a day-to-day basis is such an exciting prospect. But let's be honest. Chances are that when you're on any program, you will not be fully and continuously excited about weight loss all the time. Our desire for that sometimes wanes. That's why with this program you get more. You begin to see your weight loss in the context of valuing and expressing your entire self, and therefore you will find continual motivation and you will be committed with persistence and enthusiasm.

> To be fully alive is to be on fire with purpose.
>
> —Paramahansa Yogananda

One of my favorite things about the NutriSystem Nourish program is the support you get from the NutriSystem community. For decades, the folks at NutriSystem have been supporting people who are losing weight. Through their extensive team of counselors and weight-loss professionals, they've developed extensive skills and tools that will help you lose weight, too. Maybe you like to check in with someone when you're on a weight-loss plan. On the NutriSystem Nourish program, there's always a counselor available with whom you can talk and discuss your questions. And now you don't need to go to a weight-loss center for support. You can simply call 1-800-321-THIN, or go to www.nutrisystem.com to get the answers you need.

Or maybe you're more of a do-it-yourself dieter and just want to focus on your own plan. NutriSystem understands you, too, and offers many online services like weekly weight-loss and motivational e-classes, bulletin boards and chat rooms, an online food store for easy ordering and program management, and even a food diary for tracking your meals, all of which you can take advantage of (or not) as you see fit.

Facing Challenges

Life is a series of choices and experiences that will shape your destiny. No matter how much support you have or how motivated you are, when you are actively working on losing weight and gaining life, you will come upon these kinds of crossroads—moments when you're faced with tough decisions that take courage and conviction to make. You will constantly be met with situations that will challenge your core beliefs and require you to choose based either on fear or on faith. It is in this space that you have to ask yourself: Am I open to more—more energy, more peace, more abundance? When you make good choices—like feeding your body well, exercising, and always keeping yourself prepared and allowing the process of this program to unfold—your body will work for you. It's what it wants to do.

Challenges are inevitable, but there's one key thing you can do to overcome them: *be prepared.* A powerful way to keep your program positive and in the flow of success is to have a plan in place for the times that you know will occasionally result in a change of direction. You know, those days when life hangs a little heavier on your shoulders. When those times come—and they always do—it's a good policy to always have healthy food reserves in your freezer, fridge, cupboards, purse, and glove compartment for when the menu, buffet, or meal does not fit into your plan or busy day. And do yourself a service by removing your high-vulnerability foods from easy-access areas altogether. But perhaps more importantly, keep your mind prepared and flexible. The beauty of the NutriSystem Nourish plan is that it can be manipulated when necessary so that you can maintain control when change happens, and instead of reacting unfavorably, you will have an opportunity to grow and be creative. Your confidence will rise and your stress will fall, further benefiting your weight-loss goals.

I want you to know that the path to nourishment does not have to be about a superhuman effort to stay on plan. There will be times when you find you don't go to the gym like you said you would, or when you sneak french fries off your child's plate or even skip a meal or two. In these instances, you just have to forgive and move on. On the whole, if you surround yourself with good things—good food, good planning, and good thoughts—you can make choices that are true to yourself and live with integrity and the pride of your own accomplishments.

Excelling in the Real World

Avoid the trap of perfectionism. Often, people beginning a diet or weight-loss program feel a need to get it all *totally* right. They set their sights on not screwing up and strive to achieve the unrealistic goal of being perfect. Down this road, success rarely follows.

On this program, things will be different. Now you can let your sensibilities take a stand. Unlike other diet plans you may have tried that were extreme or promised results that quickly faded in real life, on this program you can open your heart and once again trust your body. In fact, you can hope to do far more than be perfect—you can dare to excel!

Believe in the beauty of your dreams.

—Eleanor Roosevelt

The unpredictability of life, the reality of boredom, and the issues that come with dieting and recreating your life and your relationship with food are all very real, and if you strive to master them with perfection, you'll no doubt disappoint yourself. It's true, nobody's perfect, but everyone can excel. By following this plan you will meet your nutritional needs and get your weight loss going. Then you can move on to things like living and growing your dreams. You can trust that balance will come to you, too, because it will. This program is about your own personal excellence. This is your journey. You can put yourself in a place of constant pain through continuous comparisons and competing with others (or with yourself) or you can choose to excel in your life and be free.

Commit to raising your standards. Exercise your right to choose well. And know that creating a life of genuine health and prosperity is a process, not a destination. It is a continuous commitment to daily excellence—much more than you could ever hope for from perfectionism.

Nourish for Life!

Someone once said that there are no guarantees in life. Well, I'd like to offer you this one. I guarantee that if you open up your mind and spirit to this program and invest a moderate amount of time and energy into making it work, you will find success on so many levels. Will you lose weight? *Yes!* You can lose 8 to 17 pounds in the first 4 weeks and continue losing a safe 1 to 2½ pounds each week thereafter.

Through your success, you'll finally see what a strong, powerful, and compassionate person you can be, and that's how you'll be able to take that next step and achieve long-term weight-loss management. It's all part of the evolution of you. The secret to the success of this program lies within you right now. If you connect with the part of yourself that is passionate about life, you will find success. I've seen it happen time and time again with so many patients throughout the years. By nourishing your entire self, you can achieve significant weight loss plus so much more.

Why do people fail at other diets? Because those diets are just plans for weight loss, not plans for weight loss *plus* lifelong weight management and ultimate fulfillment. You have to go for more! You are a magnificent miracle, far more than your history, more compelling than your pounds lost. You are here to be nourished in a life of happiness and purpose. You're here to evolve. And this plan will help you do just that.

The funny thing about the NutriSystem Nourish program is that while it truly offers an integrated approach to weight loss, it's actually a very simple and easy-to-follow plan built for real life and real people. You wouldn't expect that from such a well-rounded effort, but it's true. This program's beauty lies in its simplicity and applicability.

This program is the culmination of years of experience working with people just like you, conquering weight issues just like those you're facing, and it combines everything we've learned into one tangible, highly doable plan. It's all about you and helping you nourish yourself. In a world where fast food is the norm, where more is rarely seen as less and making time for yourself and your goals is virtually unheard of, the NutriSystem Nourish program stands as a beacon of light and hope for those searching for balance and simplicity in their weight-loss efforts. It's a healthy, easy-to-follow weight-loss program designed to fit you and your life so that you can reach your real and true potential.

> If you can dream it, you can do it.
>
> —Walt Disney

On this program you will lose weight. On this program you will lighten your heart. On this program you will nourish yourself from the inside out.

No matter who you are, how heavy you are, how busy you are, or how hopeless you are, you can resolve to evolve and become thinner, healthier, and happier *right now.*

It's well within your power.

Nourish!

PART FIVE

Nourishing Recipes

9

NutriSystem Nourish Recipes

Breakfast

(Order Based on Prep Time)

1. Soy Breeze
2. Mango Lassi
3. Fresh Berry and Yogurt Parfait
4. Chocolate Banana Smoothie
5. Tropical Piña Smoothie
6. Southwest Egg Scramble
7. Scrambled Eggs with Lox and Onions
8. Cheese Omelet with Salsa
9. Sunny-Side-Up Eggs and Turkey Bacon
10. Maple Granola
11. Provençal Style Frittata
12. Banana Chocolate Chip Muffins

Soy Breeze

Prep Time: 5 minutes

This smoothie is the most requested breakfast smoothie in my family.

½ large banana, sliced
1 cup soy milk, vanilla or plain
½ cup fresh or frozen strawberries
½ scoop vanilla soy protein powder*

Puree the banana, soy milk, and strawberries in a blender until smooth.

Add the protein powder and blend for 30 seconds.

Makes 1 serving.

NUTRITION INFORMATION PER SERVING

Calories: 227
Protein: 37 grams
Carbohydrate: 35 grams
Dietary Fiber: 4 grams
Fat: 4 grams
Saturated Fat: 0.1 gram
Monounsaturated Fat: 8 grams
Polyunsaturated Fat: 0.2 gram
Cholesterol: 0 milligrams
Sodium: 96 milligrams
Glycemic Index: low

Mango Lassi

Prep Time: 5 minutes

This is a great smoothie that is popular in Indian restaurants. A dash of rosewater is commonly used, but vanilla extract is a good substitute if you can't find it.

1½ cups fresh or frozen mango chunks
1½ cups low-fat or nonfat yogurt
4 ice cubes
1 tablespoon rosewater*

If using fresh mango, remove the peel and pit and cut the mango into chunks.

Puree the mango in a blender with the yogurt, ice, and rosewater until smooth.

Makes 2 servings.

*Rosewater is found in health food, gourmet, and international markets. If unavailable, use 1 teaspoon vanilla extract.

NUTRITION INFORMATION PER SERVING

Calories: 188
Protein: 10 grams
Carbohydrate: 33 grams
Dietary Fiber: 2 grams
Fat: 3 grams
Saturated Fat: 1.7 grams
Monounsaturated Fat: 0.9 gram
Polyunsaturated Fat: 0.1 gram
Cholesterol: 10 milligrams
Sodium: 122 milligrams
Glycemic Index: low

Fresh Berry and Yogurt Parfait

Prep Time: 5 minutes

This dish is colorful, fresh, and fun. Have it for dessert, too!

½ cup flavored or plain yogurt
¼ cup blueberries
2 tablespoons granola
¼ cup strawberries

Layer in a parfait glass: ¼ cup yogurt, blueberries, ¼ cup yogurt, granola, and strawberries.

Makes 1 serving.

NUTRITION INFORMATION PER SERVING

Calories: 220
Protein: 9 grams
Carbohydrate: 36 grams
Dietary Fiber: 4 grams
Fat: 5 grams
Saturated Fat: 1.3 grams
Monounsaturated Fat: 1.5 grams
Polyunsaturated Fat: 0.8 gram
Cholesterol: 6 milligrams
Sodium: 79 milligrams
Glycemic Index: low

Chocolate Banana Smoothie

Prep Time: 5 minutes

This is a delicious way to start the day.

1 large banana, peeled and cut into chunks
2 cups skim milk
1½ scoops chocolate protein powder

Puree the banana and milk in a blender until smooth. Add the protein powder and blend for 30 seconds.

Makes 2 servings. Serving size: 12 ounces.

NUTRITION INFORMATION PER SERVING

Calories: 216
Protein: 20 grams
Carbohydrate: 34 grams
Dietary Fiber: 2 grams
Fat: 0.3 gram
Saturated Fat: 0.1 gram
Monounsaturated Fat: 0 gram
Polyunsaturated Fat: 0 gram
Cholesterol: 3 milligrams
Sodium: 130 milligrams
Glycemic Index: low

Tropical Piña Smoothie

Prep Time: 5 minutes

1 cup nonfat plain yogurt
1 cup pineapple juice
½ banana, sliced
3 ice cubes
2 tablespoons fresh lime juice
1 scoop vanilla soy protein powder

Puree the yogurt, pineapple juice, banana, ice cubes, and lime juice in a blender until smooth. Add the protein powder and blend for 30 seconds.

Serve in two chilled glasses.

Makes 2 servings.

NUTRITION INFORMATION PER SERVING
Calories: 226
Protein: 15.4 grams
Carbohydrate: 42 grams
Dietary Fiber: 1 gram
Fat: 0.6 gram
Saturated Fat: 0.1 gram
Monounsaturated Fat: 2.3 grams
Polyunsaturated Fat: 0.1 gram
Cholesterol: 2.5 milligrams
Sodium: 162 milligrams
Glycemic Index: low

Southwest Egg Scramble

Prep and Cook Time: 10 minutes

3 egg whites
1 whole egg
¼ cup skim milk
pinch crushed red pepper
nonfat cooking spray or canola, peanut, safflower, or corn oil
2 tablespoons chopped onion
2 tablespoons canned and drained black beans
4 tablespoons reduced-fat grated cheddar cheese
2 tablespoons salsa

Whisk together the egg whites, egg, skim milk, and crushed pepper in a bowl. Spray a nonstick frying pan with nonfat cooking spray or lightly coat with oil. Heat the pan to medium heat, add onion, and sauté for 1 minute. Add the egg mixture to the pan, stirring continuously to scramble. Add black beans and grated cheese; finish cooking eggs to desired consistency.

Serve on individual plates and top each portion with 1 ablespoon salsa.

Makes 2 servings.

NUTRITION INFORMATION PER SERVING
Calories: 121
Protein: 14 grams
Carbohydrate: 6.8 grams
Dietary Fiber: 0.9 gram
Fat: 4 grams
Saturated Fat: 1.5 grams
Monounsaturated Fat: 1.4 grams
Polyunsaturated Fat: 0.4 gram
Cholesterol: 126 milligrams
Sodium: 311 milligrams
Glycemic Index: low

Scrambled Eggs with Lox and Onions

Prep and Cook Time: 10 minutes

This is a simple and flavorful breakfast dish. Lox is smoked salmon. Use Nova Scotia, if possible, because it is less salty.

2 whole eggs
¼ cup egg whites or liquid egg replacement product
1 tablespoon skim milk
1 teaspoon canola, peanut, safflower, or corn oil
½ medium onion, peeled and chopped
1 ounce lox, preferably Nova Scotia, cut into thin strips
freshly ground pepper

Combine the eggs, egg whites or liquid egg replacement product, and milk in a bowl by whisking together with a fork. Heat the oil in a nonstick skillet. Cook the onion and lox together for a minute, then add the egg mixture to the pan. Stir and cook to desired consistency. Sprinkle with some freshly ground black pepper.

Makes 2 servings.

NUTRITION INFORMATION PER SERVING
Calories: 156
Protein: 14 grams
Carbohydrate: 5 grams
Dietary Fiber: 1 gram
Fat: 9 grams
Saturated Fat: 2 grams
Monounsaturated Fat: 4 grams
Polyunsaturated Fat: 2 grams
Cholesterol: 250 milligrams
Sodium: 424 milligrams
Glycemic Index: low

Cheese Omelet with Salsa

Prep and Cook Time: 10 minutes

This omelet is easy, light, and low in calories.

1 whole egg
4 egg whites
¼ cup skim milk
1 tablespoon chopped parsley
freshly ground pepper
1 teaspoon canola, peanut, safflower, or corn oil
1 ounce cheese, such as cheddar, American, Swiss, or Muenster
¼ cup salsa

NUTRITION INFORMATION PER SERVING
Calories: 154
Protein: 15 grams
Carbohydrate: 5 grams
Dietary Fiber: 0 gram
Fat: 7 grams
Saturated Fat: 3 grams
Monounsaturated Fat: 1 gram
Polyunsaturated Fat: 0.4 gram
Cholesterol: 139 milligrams
Sodium: 368 milligrams
Glycemic Index: low

Cheese Omelet with Salsa (continued)

Using a fork or whisk, mix the egg, egg whites, milk, parsley, and ground pepper in a bowl. Lightly oil a nonstick frying pan. Heat pan on medium, then pour in the egg mixture. Cook for about 3 minutes, occasionally lifting the sides of the omelet to let the uncooked egg seep underneath. When the egg is about three-quarters cooked, put the cheese on top. Flip one-half of the omelet over the other half and cook 1 more minute.

Serve with 2 tablespoons of salsa on top.

Makes 2 servings.

Sunny-Side-Up Eggs and Turkey Bacon

Cook Time: 10 minutes

Turkey bacon is leaner than pork bacon and has great flavor. Health food stores sell a nitrite-free type, which will not last as long but is better for you.

1 egg
2 strips turkey bacon, nitrite-free if possible
nonfat cooking spray or canola, peanut, safflower, or
   corn oil

Lightly oil a nonstick frying pan or griddle, or spray with nonstick spray.

Cook bacon strips in the pan for 1 minute on each side. Move to the edge of the pan and crack the egg into the center. Cook the egg until the yolk is no longer runny.

Makes 1 serving.

NUTRITION INFORMATION PER SERVING
Calories: 156
Protein: 12 grams
Carbohydrate: 1 gram
Dietary Fiber: 0 gram
Fat: 12 grams
Saturated Fat: 3 grams
Monounsaturated Fat: 4 grams
Polyunsaturated Fat: 2 grams
Cholesterol: 272 milligrams
Sodium: 412 milligrams
Glycemic Index: low

Maple Granola

Prep Time: 5 minutes
Cook Time: 15 minutes

2 cups old-fashioned oats
¼ cup wheat germ
2 tablespoons hulled sunflower seeds
1 teaspoon ground cinnamon
2 tablespoons canola or safflower oil
2 tablespoons maple syrup
1 teaspoon vanilla extract
2 tablespoons raisins

NUTRITION
INFORMATION PER
SERVING
Calories: 181
Protein: 5.5 grams
Carbohydrate: 25 grams
Dietary Fiber: 4 grams
Fat: 7 grams
Saturated Fat: 0.8 gram
Monounsaturated Fat: 2
   grams
Polyunsaturated Fat: 1.3
   grams
Cholesterol: 0 milligram
Sodium: 3 milligrams
Glycemic Index: low

Preheat oven to 350 degrees. Spread the oats on a baking sheet and bake for 10 minutes.

Remove from the oven and transfer to a bowl. (Do not turn off the oven.) Add the wheat germ, sunflower seeds, and cinnamon to the bowl.

In a separate bowl, mix the oil, maple syrup, and vanilla together. Pour this mixture over the oat mixture. Stir to coat. Add the raisins.

Spread this mixture back onto the baking pan. Bake for 5 minutes. Let cool. Store in a plastic bag or glass jar.

Makes 8 servings. Serving size: ½ cup.

Provençal Style Frittata

Prep Time: 5 minutes
Cook Time: 15 minutes

This version of a frittata is an omelet flipped over into a second pan. You can change the types of ingredients to change the flavors.

NUTRITION INFORMATION PER SERVING

Calories: 173
Protein: 15 grams
Carbohydrate: 3 grams
Dietary Fiber: 0.5 gram
Fat: 11 grams
Saturated Fat: 6 grams
Monounsaturated Fat: 3 grams
Polyunsaturated Fat: 0.8 gram
Cholesterol: 202 milligrams
Sodium: 405 milligrams
Glycemic Index: low

3 eggs
¾ cup egg whites or liquid egg replacement product
¼ cup chopped fresh basil or spinach
2 tablespoons chopped sun-dried tomatoes or fresh
    tomato slices
3 ounces goat cheese, crumbled fine
¼ teaspoon salt
freshly ground pepper to taste
1 teaspoon canola, peanut, safflower, or corn oil

Combine the eggs and egg whites or egg replacement product in a bowl. Add the basil or spinach, sun-dried tomatoes, goat cheese, salt, and pepper to the eggs. Lightly oil a nonstick frying pan and heat on medium. Add the egg mixture to the pan, cooking until edges are done and middle is almost done.

Heat a second nonstick frying pan that is lightly coated with oil over medium heat. Flip the frittata over into the second heated pan. Cook 1 to 2 minutes.

Makes 4 servings.

Banana Chocolate Chip Muffins

Prep Time: 15 minutes
Cook Time: 25 minutes

These muffins are a tasty way to start the day or use them for snacks or desserts. They freeze well: wrap in foil or place muffins in a suitable freezer container or plastic bag.

2 tablespoons canola or safflower oil
½ cup brown sugar
1 egg
1 egg white
1 cup mashed banana (2 ripe medium bananas, mashed)
1 cup skim milk or nonfat buttermilk
1½ cups whole-wheat flour
½ cup gluten flour
1 teaspoon baking powder
1 teaspoon baking soda
½ teaspoon salt
2 teaspoons cinnamon
¼ cup semisweet chocolate chips

NUTRITION INFORMATION PER SERVING

Calories: 179
Protein: 5 grams
Carbohydrate: 31 grams
Dietary Fiber: 3 grams
Fat: 5 grams
Saturated Fat: 1 gram
Monounsaturated Fat: 1.6 grams
Polyunsaturated Fat: 0.8 gram
Cholesterol: 21 milligrams
Sodium: 259 milligrams
Glycemic Index: low–medium

Preheat oven to 350 degrees. Lightly oil each section of a 12-section muffin tin. Mix the oil and sugar together in a bowl until smooth. Add the egg, egg white, banana, and milk. Mix well.

In a separate bowl, mix all the dry ingredients together. Then combine the liquid and dry ingredients, stirring until lump-free. Spoon the mixture into the muffin tin. Bake 20 to 22 minutes.

Makes 12 muffins.

Lunch

(Order Based on Prep Time)

1. Baked Tofu "Chef's Salad"
2. Open-Faced Turkey Reuben Sandwich
3. Turkey Roll-Up
4. Smoked Salmon Wrap
5. Antipasto Salad with Tuna
6. Tuscan White Bean Salad with Tuna
7. Black Bean Gazpacho
8. Vegetable Quesadilla
9. Mexican Black Bean Salad with Salsa
10. Tuna Salad Niçoise
11. Vegetable Miso Soup
12. Layered Mexican Egg Pie
13. Salmon Corn Chowder
14. Curried Butternut Squash Soup
15. Crustless Quiche Lorraine
16. Cobb Salad
17. Chicken Salad with Grapes
18. Savory Lentil Soup

Baked Tofu Chef's Salad

Prep Time: 5 minutes (using prepared baked tofu)

Baked tofu is sold in health food stores in a variety of flavors. You can easily make it yourself with the recipe below. It is a satisfying food rich in protein.

2 cups chopped lettuce greens
3 ounces baked tofu* cut into bite-size pieces
3 ounces baby carrots (7 average-size baby carrots)
1 medium tomato, cored and chopped
low-fat salad dressing of your choice

NUTRITION INFORMATION PER SERVING

Calories: 270
Protein: 17 grams
Carbohydrate: 33 grams
Dietary Fiber: 8 grams
Fat: 8 grams
Saturated Fat: 1.5 grams
Monounsaturated Fat: 0 gram
Polyunsaturated Fat: 0.2 gram
Cholesterol: 0 milligram
Sodium: 720 milligrams
Glycemic Index: low

Place the lettuce on a dinner plate. Top with the remaining ingredients.

Homemade Baked Tofu*

1 pound extra-firm fresh tofu
⅓ cup teriyaki sauce (store-bought, or homemade, see recipe below)**

Preheat oven to 350 degrees. Cut the tofu into slices about ½ inch thick. Place in a bowl and carefully mix with the teriyaki sauce. Lay foil or parchment paper on a baking pan. Lay the tofu on top, spoon a little extra sauce on each piece, and bake 20 minutes.

Homemade Teriyaki**

⅓ cup low-sodium soy sauce
1 tablespoon fructose
½ teaspoon fresh chopped ginger

Heat the soy sauce, fructose, and ginger in a pan on low heat for about 3 minutes to mix the flavors and dissolve the fructose.

Makes 1 serving.

Open-Faced Turkey Reuben Sandwich

Prep and Cook Time: 5 minutes

You can make this sandwich with either turkey pastrami or very lean corned beef.

NUTRITION INFORMATION PER SERVING

Calories: 204
Protein: 20 grams
Carbohydrate: 16 grams
Dietary Fiber: 1.4 grams
Fat: 6 grams
Saturated Fat: 2.4 grams
Monounsaturated Fat:
  0.3 gram
Polyunsaturated Fat: 0.1
  gram
Cholesterol: 49
  milligrams
Sodium: 897 milligrams
Glycemic Index: low

    1 slice rye bread or pumpernickel bread
    1 teaspoon light mayonnaise
    1 teaspoon ketchup
    2 ounces turkey pastrami or lean corned beef
    2 tablespoons sauerkraut
    ¾ ounce thinly sliced Swiss cheese or Jarlsberg, reduced-fat and low-sodium if possible

Preheat broiler or toaster oven to broil. Lay the bread on a baking pan. Mix the light mayonnaise and ketchup together in a bowl. Spread this mixture on top of the bread. Lay the pastrami or corned beef on top of the bread. Spoon 2 tablespoons of sauerkraut on top of the meat. Top with sliced cheese. Broil until the cheese melts.

Makes 1 serving.

Turkey Roll-Up

Prep Time: 10 minutes

Simple and easy. Dress it up with your favorite cheese, some variety of turkey, and specialty mustards. Basil or other herbs add great flavor.

NUTRITION INFORMATION PER SERVING

Calories: 234
Protein: 19 grams
Carbohydrate: 19 grams
Dietary Fiber: 2 grams
Fat: 10 grams
Saturated Fat: 2.6 grams
Monounsaturated Fat: 0
  gram
Polyunsaturated Fat: 0
  gram
Cholesterol: 32
  milligrams
Sodium: 188 milligrams
Glycemic Index: low

    ½ ounce sliced Muenster, Swiss, or American cheese, reduced fat and low sodium, if possible
    1 tortilla, whole-wheat chapati or whole-wheat flat bread wrap
    2 ounces sliced turkey
    prepared mustard
    fresh basil or lettuce
    fresh sliced tomato

Lay the cheese on top of the tortilla, chapati, or flat bread wrap. Heat in the microwave for 20 seconds at high heat. Lay the turkey on top and all around. Spread some mustard to your liking on top of the turkey. Lay the basil or lettuce and tomato on top. Wrap in a tight roll from one end to the other. (If brown bagging for lunch, secure with toothpicks and wrap tightly in plastic wrap.)

Makes 1 serving.

Smoked Salmon Wrap

Prep Time: 10 minutes

Delicious and easy, this is like lox and bagels without the heavy bagel.

One 11-inch wrap or tortilla, preferably whole-wheat
1 ounce light cream cheese (about 2 tablespoons)
2 ounces Nova Scotia smoked salmon lox or 3 ounces kippered salmon
4 thin slices cucumber
2 slices fresh tomato
2 leaves lettuce, washed and dried
⅛ red onion, peeled and sliced very thin
½ teaspoon dried dill or 1 teaspoon fresh chopped dill

NUTRITION INFORMATION PER SERVING
Calories: 157
Protein: 10 grams
Carbohydrate: 18.5 grams
Dietary Fiber: 1.4 grams
Fat: 4.6 grams
Saturated Fat: 1.8 grams
Monounsaturated Fat: 1.3 grams
Polyunsaturated Fat: 4 grams
Cholesterol: 15 milligrams
Sodium: 500 milligrams
Glycemic Index: low

Lay the wrap or tortilla open on a plate. Spread the cream cheese all around the top of the wrap. Lay the smoked or kippered salmon on top of the cream cheese. Lay the cucumber, tomato, and lettuce on top of the salmon. Sprinkle with red onion slices and dill. Roll the wrap or tortilla tightly from one end to the other. Cut in half. Wrap each half tightly in plastic to brown-bag.

Makes 2 servings.

Antipasto Salad with Tuna

Prep Time: 10 minutes

This salad is easy to put together and full of flavor.

NUTRITION INFORMATION PER SERVING

Calories: 290
Protein: 32 grams
Carbohydrate: 18 grams
Dietary Fiber: 3 grams
Fat: 10 grams
Saturated Fat: 4 grams
Monounsaturated Fat: 4 grams
Polyunsaturated Fat: 2 grams
Cholesterol: 48 milligrams
Sodium: 750 milligrams
Glycemic Index: low

6 cups lettuce leaves
4 roasted red peppers, packed in water and drained, or fresh roasted peppers
3 ounces fresh mozzarella balls, cut into large chunks
16 small black olives, drained
¼ cup fresh basil leaves, chopped
½ cup canned chickpeas (garbanzo beans), drained
15-ounce can water-packed artichoke hearts, drained
1 12-ounce can tuna (white albacore, in water), drained
low-fat Italian salad dressing

Lay the lettuce leaves on a platter. Top with roasted red peppers, mozzarella, olives, basil, chickpeas, artichoke hearts, and tuna. Serve with a low-fat Italian dressing.

Makes 4 servings.

Tuscan White Bean Salad with Tuna

Prep Time: 10 minutes

This is a filling lunch salad or light dinner. Substitute sardines for tuna if you prefer. Serve alone or on a bed of washed greens.

NUTRITION INFORMATION PER SERVING

Calories: 222
Protein: 16 grams
Carbohydrate: 23 grams
Dietary Fiber: 6 grams
Fat: 7.5 grams
Saturated Fat: 1 gram
Monounsaturated Fat: 4.4 grams
Polyunsaturated Fat: 1.4 grams
Cholesterol: 18 milligrams
Sodium: 689 milligrams
Glycemic Index: low

3 cups broccoli florets
¼ cup chopped red onion
2 ripe tomatoes, cored and chopped
15-ounce can white beans, rinsed, or 1½ cups cooked white beans
¼ cup chopped basil
6-ounce can tuna (white albacore, in water), drained, or 6 ounces fresh cooked tuna, crumbled
1 teaspoon fresh chopped rosemary

Dressing

1½ tablespoons olive oil
2 tablespoons lemon juice
1 tablespoon vinegar
1½ teaspoons honey mustard
¼ teaspoon salt
pinch red pepper flakes

Steam or microwave the broccoli for 2 minutes, making sure it stays bright and crisp. Combine the onion, tomatoes, white beans, basil, tuna, and rosemary in a bowl. Add the broccoli. Mix together the dressing ingredients in a separate bowl. Stir into the salad.

Makes 4 servings.

Black Bean Gazpacho

Prep Time: 15 minutes

This version of the refreshing cold soup has black beans. They are puréed, so you can't see them, but they add both flavor and protein. Have a 12-ounce portion for lunch or a 6-ounce portion as a snack.

1 clove garlic, peeled
1 cucumber, peeled, seeded, and cut into chunks
1 green bell or poblano pepper, seeded
½ medium avocado, peeled and seeded
2 fresh ripe tomatoes, cored, or 15-ounce can diced tomatoes
2 tablespoons fresh parsley
1½ teaspoons chili powder
3 scallions
4 cups low-sodium tomato juice
1 can black beans (about 1½ cups)
½ teaspoon salt

NUTRITION INFORMATION PER SERVING
Calories: 170
Protein: 12 grams
Carbohydrate: 23 grams
Dietary Fiber: 6.2 grams
Fat: 4.5 grams
Saturated Fat: 0.6 gram
Monounsaturated Fat: 2 grams
Polyunsaturated Fat: 1 gram
Cholesterol: 0 milligram
Sodium: 534 milligrams
Glycemic Index: low

Place all ingredients in a food processor or blender. Purée for about 20 seconds; stop. Purée again for 20

Black Bean Gazpacho (continued)

seconds; stop. Continue until mixture looks like a chunky soup. Check to make sure there are no large pieces of vegetable left.

Serve in chilled bowls. Garnish with fresh scallions if you like.

Makes 6 servings. Serving size: 12 ounces.

Vegetable Quesadilla

Prep and Cook Time: 15 minutes

Easy and delicious! This can be reheated in the microwave for 1 minute if you brown-bag.

½ green pepper, seeded and sliced
¼ onion, peeled and sliced
¼ cup salsa (mild, medium, or hot, depending on your taste)
¾ ounce grated cheddar cheese
1 whole-wheat chapati or tortilla
½ teaspoon canola, peanut, safflower, or corn oil

NUTRITION INFORMATION PER SERVING

Calories: 250
Protein: 9 grams
Carbohydrate: 26 grams
Dietary Fiber: 2.2 grams
Fat: 12 grams
Saturated Fat: 5 grams
Monounsaturated Fat: 1.4 grams
Polyunsaturated Fat: 0.8 gram
Cholesterol: 23 milligrams
Sodium: 727 milligrams
Glycemic Index: low

Cook the green pepper and onion slices in a nonstick pan with 2 tablespoons of the salsa for a few minutes until the vegetables wilt. Remove vegetables from the pan. Place the cheese on half of the tortilla, then top with the sautéed vegetables. Flip the other half of the tortilla over the vegetables.

Heat the oil in the nonstick skillet, then cook the quesadilla for 1 to 2 minutes on each side to melt the cheese. Transfer the quesadilla from the pan to a plate. Cut into thirds. Top with the remaining salsa.

Makes 1 serving.

Mexican Black Bean Salad with Salsa

Prep and Cook Time: 25 minutes (using canned beans)

Poblano chilis look like elongated dark green bell peppers. They are spicier than green peppers with a wonderful flavor. If you can't find them, use a chopped jalapeño pepper instead.

NUTRITION INFORMATION PER SERVING

Calories: 191
Protein: 9 grams
Carbohydrate: 40 grams
Dietary Fiber: 11 grams
Fat: 4 grams
Saturated Fat: 0.5 gram
Monounsaturated Fat: 2.4 grams
Polyunsaturated Fat: 0.6 gram
Cholesterol: 0 milligram
Sodium: 667 milligrams
Glycemic Index: low

1 tablespoon canola, peanut, safflower, or corn oil

2 cloves garlic, peeled and chopped

½ poblano chili, seeded and chopped

½ red bell pepper, seeded and chopped

1 cup canned corn kernels, drained

1 tablespoon chili powder

two 15-ounce cans black beans, drained (about 3 cups), or 1 pound dried beans, cooked (see directions below*)

juice of 3 limes

½ cup red salsa

¼ cup red onion, peeled and chopped

½ teaspoon salt

¼ cup chopped fresh cilantro (coriander leaves)

1 head of lettuce, leaves washed and left whole or halved

Heat oil and garlic in a frying pan. Add the poblano pepper, red bell pepper, corn kernels, and chili powder. Cook 5 minutes until peppers are soft. Remove from heat.

In a bowl, combine the sautéed vegetable mixture, beans, lime juice, salsa, onion, salt, and cilantro. Serve on top of the lettuce.

Makes 5 servings. Serving size: 1 cup.

*To cook beans from scratch: Pick through the beans, looking to remove any pebbles or pieces of dirt. Rinse. Bring 1 quart of water and raw beans to a boil and boil 1 minute. Remove from heat and let sit 1 hour. Drain beans, then refill the pot with water, bring to a boil, reduce to a simmer, and cook 30 minutes or until beans are soft.

Tuna Salad Niçoise

Prep Time: 15 minutes
Cook Time: 15 minutes

Niçoise olives are tiny black olives. If you use canned olives instead, use half the amount.

NUTRITION
INFORMATION PER
SERVING
Calories: 290
Protein: 30 grams
Carbohydrate: 18 grams
Dietary Fiber: 7 grams
Fat: 11 grams
Saturated Fat: 2.5 grams
Monounsaturated Fat: 4
    grams
Polyunsaturated Fat: 3
    grams
Cholesterol: 164
    milligrams
Sodium: 1,006 milligrams
Glycemic Index: low

3 cups romaine lettuce leaves, torn into bite-size pieces

2 hard-boiled eggs, peeled and chopped

1 cucumber, peeled and sliced

¼ pound green beans, steamed or microwaved for 3 minutes

¼ pound cherry tomatoes or other ripe tomatoes, cut into chunks

1 ounce niçoise olives with pits (30 olives)

4 anchovies

6-ounce can tuna (white albacore, in water), drained

Dressing

3 tablespoons low-fat salad dressing

½ teaspoon prepared mustard

1 tablespoon chopped parsley

½ teaspoon fresh or ¼ teaspoon dried dill

Divide the lettuce between two dinner plates. Arrange all of the salad ingredients on top of the lettuce, sprinkling the tuna on top.

Combine dressing ingredients in a small bowl and stir until mixed. Top each salad with 2 tablespoons of the salad dressing or another low-fat dressing of your choice.

Makes 2 servings.

Vegetable Miso Soup

Prep Time: 20 minutes
Cook Time: 15 minutes

Miso is Japanese fermented bean paste. Added to soup broth, it adds both great flavor and good nutrition. This soup is easy to make and filling. Serve it by itself or serve four 1-cup servings with a little cooked brown rice.

NUTRITION INFORMATION PER SERVING

Calories: 271
Protein: 21 grams
Carbohydrate: 22 grams
Dietary Fiber: 6 grams
Fat: 12 grams
Saturated Fat: 2 grams
Monounsaturated Fat: 2.1 grams
Polyunsaturated Fat: 4 grams
Cholesterol: 3 milligrams
Sodium: 958 milligrams
Glycemic Index: low

½ tablespoon toasted sesame oil
2 slices ginger, peeled and chopped fine
2 garlic cloves, peeled and chopped fine
1 medium onion, cut in half and sliced into thin strips
2 medium carrots, sliced in ½-inch-thick diagonals
3 cups vegetable stock, or defatted unsalted chicken stock
1 cup chopped Swiss chard, cabbage, or spinach
1 cup broccoli florets
6 ounces tofu cut into 1-inch cubes (or baked tofu)
1 tablespoon miso paste*
freshly ground pepper to taste

In a 2-quart soup pot, cook oil, ginger, garlic, onion, and carrots together for about 5 minutes. Add the soup stock and cook 5 minutes on low heat. Add the Swiss chard (or other greens), broccoli, and tofu. Simmer 5 minutes on low.

Remove ½ cup of the stock and mix it with the miso in a measuring cup. Stir until lumps dissolve. Return the miso mixture to the soup. Season with pepper and cook 1 more minute.

Makes 2 servings. Serving size: 2 cups.

*Miso is found in health food or Asian markets. There are many varieties, each with a different flavor. Keep refrigerated after opening.

Layered Mexican Egg Pie

Prep Time: 10 minutes
Cook Time: 30 minutes

This is really easy and looks as if you worked hard to make it. The ingredients combine and provide a lot of flavor. It's a great breakfast or brunch dish, too.

3 eggs
½ cup egg whites or liquid egg replacement product
1 cup red or green chili salsa (mild, medium, or hot, depending on your preference)
two 8-inch whole-wheat tortillas or chapatis
3 ounces cheddar cheese, grated
½ small zucchini, thinly sliced
1 green chili, canned or fresh, cut into strips
1 teaspoon ground chili pepper

NUTRITION INFORMATION PER SERVING

Calories: 245
Protein: 18 grams
Carbohydrate: 13 grams
Dietary Fiber: 0.5 gram
Fat: 13 grams
Saturated Fat: 5 grams
Monounsaturated Fat: 1.7 grams
Polyunsaturated Fat: 0.6 gram
Cholesterol: 207 milligrams
Sodium: 711 milligrams
Glycemic Index: low

Preheat the oven to 350 degrees. Mix the eggs and egg whites or egg replacement product together in a bowl.

Oil an 8-inch pie pan or spray it with nonstick cooking spray. Spoon ½ cup of salsa on the bottom of the pan to cover lightly. Top with a whole-wheat tortilla or chapati. Sprinkle half of the grated cheese on top. Pour half of the egg mixture over the cheese. Lay another tortilla on top. Spread the remaining salsa on the tortilla. Top with the remaining grated cheese. Lay zucchini slices on top. Pour the remaining egg mixture over the pie. Lay chili strips around the top. Sprinkle chili pepper on top.

Bake for 25 to 30 minutes or until center is slightly firm to touch.

Makes 4 servings.

Salmon Corn Chowder

Prep Time: 20 minutes
Cook Time: 20 minutes

This creamy soup is perfect for a cold day. You can substitute cooked chicken for the salmon if you prefer.

NUTRITION INFORMATION PER SERVING

Calories: 157
Protein: 15 grams
Carbohydrate: 13 grams
Dietary Fiber: 1.4 grams
Fat: 5 grams
Saturated Fat: 0.8 gram
Monounsaturated Fat: 2.2 grams
Polyunsaturated Fat: 1.4 grams
Cholesterol: 26 milligrams
Sodium: 538 milligrams
Glycemic Index: low

4 garlic cloves, peeled and chopped
1 medium onion, peeled and chopped
1 tablespoon canola, peanut, safflower, or corn oil
1 cup chopped celery
3½ cups fresh corn kernels, or 1 pound frozen corn kernels
½ pound small red new potatoes, cut into chunks
3 cups vegetable or fish stock (broth), unsalted
½ red bell pepper, seeded and chopped
12 ounces evaporated skim milk
12 ounces canned salmon, skinned and boned, or fresh cooked salmon, skinned and boned
1 tablespoon chili pepper
1½ teaspoons salt (use less salt if using canned salmon)

In a soup pot, sauté the garlic and onion in the oil for 2 minutes. Add the celery, corn kernels, potatoes, and stock. Cook for 10 minutes on medium heat. Add the red bell pepper and evaporated milk. Cook on low heat for a few more minutes or until the potato chunks are fork-tender.

Purée half the soup in a blender. Return blended soup to the pot.

If using fresh salmon, break the salmon into smaller chunks. If using canned salmon, remove the skin and larger round bones. Add to the soup. Add the chili pepper and salt. Cook a few more minutes.

Makes 10 servings.

Curried Butternut Squash Soup

Prep Time: 15 minutes
Cook Time: 25 minutes

This recipe can be doubled and it freezes well. It is a great source of vitamin A.

NUTRITION
INFORMATION PER
SERVING

Calories: 133
Protein: 7 grams
Carbohydrate: 28 grams
Dietary Fiber: 6 grams
Fat: 0.4 gram
Saturated Fat: 0.1 gram
Monounsaturated Fat:
  0.1 gram
Polyunsaturated Fat: 0.1
  gram
Cholesterol: 3 milligrams
Sodium: 337 milligrams
Glycemic Index: low

2 pounds butternut squash
1 medium onion, peeled and chopped
2 garlic cloves, peeled and chopped
4 cups water
1 vegetable or chicken bouillon cube*
1½ to 2 teaspoons curry powder
12-ounce can evaporated skim milk
freshly ground pepper to taste

Cut the squash in half; remove the seeds and cut the squash into chunks. In a soup pot, cook the onion, garlic, and butternut chunks with the water, bouillon cube, and curry powder for about 20 minutes or until squash is tender. Remove squash and carefully peel skin off. Return the peeled squash to the pot. Add the milk. Purée soup in batches in the blender. Add pepper and taste for seasoning.

Makes 6 servings.

*Homemade vegetable stock or chicken stock is even better. Use 4 cups stock instead of the 1 bouillon cube and 4 cups water. If stock is not salted, you may need to add more salt to the soup according to your taste.

Crustless Quiche Lorraine

Prep Time: 15 minutes
Cook Time: 30 minutes

Turkey bacon is lower in fat than regular bacon and tastes great. Combined with leeks and Swiss cheese, it makes a filling and satisfying lunch.

2 strips turkey bacon
1 leek, ends trimmed, white stalk chopped
3 eggs
¾ cup egg whites or liquid egg replacement product
12-ounce can evaporated skim milk
1 cup grated Swiss cheese
¼ teaspoon ground black pepper
1 medium zucchini, sliced

NUTRITION INFORMATION PER SERVING

Calories: 174
Protein: 15 grams
Carbohydrate: 10 grams
Dietary Fiber: 0.3 gram
Fat: 8 grams
Saturated Fat: 4 grams
Monounsaturated Fat: 0.8 gram
Polyunsaturated Fat: 0.6 gram
Cholesterol: 142 milligrams
Sodium: 247 milligrams
Glycemic Index: low

Preheat oven to 350 degrees. In a nonstick frying pan, cook the turkey bacon for 1 minute on each side over medium heat. Remove bacon from pan. Add the chopped leek and cook with 2 tablespoons water for 2 to 3 minutes. Turn off heat and set aside.

Combine the eggs, egg whites or egg replacement product, milk, Swiss cheese, and black pepper in a bowl. Crumble up the bacon into small pieces and add the bacon and leeks to the bowl. Lightly oil a pie plate. Line the bottom of the pie pan with zucchini. Top with the egg mixture. Bake for 25 minutes.

Makes 6 servings.

Cobb Salad

Prep Time: 20 minutes
Cook Time: 30 minutes

This is a popular salad served in many restaurants and it is filled with flavor and texture.

1 head of Bibb lettuce torn into bite-size pieces
2 ripe tomatoes cut into chunks
1 ripe avocado, peeled, seeded, and sliced
2 hard boiled-eggs, peeled and chopped
2 strips turkey bacon, cooked and chopped fine
8 pitted black olives
1 cup corn kernels, fresh steamed if possible
8 ounces grilled, poached, or canned chunk chicken or deli turkey, sliced into strips
¼ cup crumbled blue cheese (this is traditional, but use only if you like blue cheese)
low-fat dressing of your choice

Divide the lettuce on each of 4 plates. Arrange the other ingredients on top of the lettuce.

Serve with your favorite low-fat salad dressing.

Makes 4 salads.

NUTRITION INFORMATION PER SERVING

Calories: 267
Protein: 17 grams
Carbohydrate: 15 grams
Dietary Fiber: 3.8 grams
Fat: 17 grams
Saturated Fat: 4 grams
Monounsaturated Fat: 6.6 grams
Polyunsaturated Fat: 2 grams
Cholesterol: 157 milligrams
Sodium: 323 milligrams
Glycemic Index: low

Chicken Salad with Grapes

Prep Time: 15 minutes
Cook Time: 1 hour (using fresh chicken)

A simple variation on a popular recipe.

4 pounds fresh fryer chicken
½ cup reduced-fat mayonnaise
1 cup green seedless grapes
freshly ground pepper to taste

Bring 2 quarts of water to a boil, then reduce to a simmer. Add the chicken and cook on low for 1 hour. Remove the chicken from the cooking liquid, saving the liquid as a soup stock for other recipes. Let the chicken

NUTRITION INFORMATION PER SERVING

Calories: 186
Protein: 16 grams
Carbohydrate: 6.4 grams
Dietary Fiber: 0.3 gram
Fat: 10.5 grams
Saturated Fat: 2 grams
Monounsaturated Fat: 1.4 grams
Polyunsaturated Fat: 0.9 gram
Cholesterol: 54 milligrams
Sodium: 199 milligrams
Glycemic Index: low

cool. When the chicken is cool enough to touch, remove the meat from the bone, discarding the skin and bones. Shred chicken into bite-size pieces. Combine the chicken meat, mayonnaise, and grapes in a bowl. Season with pepper.

Makes 6 servings.

Savory Lentil Soup

Prep Time: 20 minutes
Cook Time: 1 hour

This soup is great on a cold fall or winter day for lunch or dinner. It freezes well and lasts about 3 to 4 days refrigerated.

NUTRITION INFORMATION PER SERVING

Calories: 171
Protein: 5.2 grams
Carbohydrate: 32 grams
Dietary Fiber: 6 grams
Fat: 4 grams
Saturated Fat: 0.6 gram
Monounsaturated Fat: 2.7 grams
Polyunsaturated Fat: 0.6 gram
Cholesterol: 4 milligrams
Sodium: 401 milligrams
Glycemic Index: low

1 tablespoon oil
1 medium onion, peeled and chopped
3 garlic cloves, peeled and chopped
2 raw strips turkey bacon, nitrite-free if possible, chopped
5 medium carrots, peeled if necessary and cut into chunks
3 stalks celery, chopped
3 green peppers, seeded and chopped
1 pound lentils, rinsed
2 small sweet potatoes, peeled and cubed
3 bay leaves
sprig of thyme
sprig of rosemary
1 bouillon cube (chicken, beef, or vegetable)
13 cups water
2 teaspoons grated lemon peel
3 ounces tomato paste

Heat the oil in a large soup pot. Add the onion, garlic, and turkey bacon and sauté for 3 minutes. Add the carrots, celery, green pepper, lentils, sweet potatoes, bay leaves, thyme, rosemary, bouillon cube, and water. Cook for 45 minutes, stirring occasionally. Add the lemon peel and tomato paste and cook another 10 minutes .

Makes 6 servings. Serving size: 16 ounces.

Dinner

(Order Based on Prep Time)

1. Chicken Caesar Salad
2. Pan-Seared Trout with Pine Nuts and Pumpkin Seeds
3. Curried Chickpea Stew with Spinach
4. Teriyaki Swordfish with Sugar Snap Peas and Portobello Mushrooms
5. Spinach Strawberry Salad with Goat Cheese and Chicken
6. Sunflower Burgers
7. Grilled Catfish with Tomato Cilantro Sauce
8. Turkey Tostadas
9. Picadillo
10. Tilapia with Honey Mustard Sauce
11. Sautéed Peppers and Onions with Turkey Sausage
12. Salmon in BBQ Sauce with Waldorf Salad
13. Vegetarian Chili
14. Chicken Cacciatore
15. Mussels Marinara
16. Shrimp in Thai Red Curry Sauce
17. Cheese Ravioli with Tomato Basil Sauce
18. Black Bean Stew
19. Spinach Mushroom Crepes
20. Southwestern Meatloaf
21. Teriyaki Beef and Broccoli
22. Grilled Ratatouille with Shrimp or Tofu
23. Eggplant Parmesan
24. Marinated Asian Beef Salad
25. Turkey London Broil
26. Beef Stew
27. Chicken Kabobs with Dates
28. Shepherd's Pie
29. Chicken with Cabbage in Spicy Peanut Dressing
30. Thai Chicken with Broccoli
31. Arroz Con Pollo

Chicken Caesar Salad

Prep Time: 15 minutes

Salad dressing

2 garlic cloves, peeled and crushed

juice of 1 lemon

1 teaspoon prepared mustard

2–3 teaspoons chopped anchovies, depending on taste

2 teaspoons oil from anchovy can, or olive oil

½ teaspoon Worcestershire sauce

3 tablespoons liquid egg replacement product

Salad

4 cups romaine lettuce

8 ounces cooked chicken (from a boiled or roasted chicken, poached or grilled chicken breast, sliced), skin removed

2 tablespoons Parmesan cheese

2 tablespoons pine nuts or toasted sliced almonds

NUTRITION INFORMATION PER SERVING

Calories: 400
Protein: 54 grams
Carbohydrate: 10 grams
Dietary Fiber: 3.3 grams
Fat: 16 grams
Saturated Fat: 3 grams
Monounsaturated Fat: 4.6 grams
Polyunsaturated Fat: 3.7 grams
Cholesterol: 121 milligrams
Sodium: 894 milligrams
Glycemic Index: low

Combine the salad dressing ingredients in a blender, food processor, or with a mortar and pestle.

Tear the lettuce into bite-size pieces. Toss the greens with the dressing. Separate onto two plates. Top with the cooked chicken.

Sprinkle Parmesan cheese on top of each salad, then sprinkle pine nuts on top of each.

Makes 2 servings.

Pan-Seared Trout with Pine Nuts and Pumpkin Seeds

Prep Time: 5 minutes
Cook Time: 10 minutes

This is a wonderful dish, full of flavor and easy to make.

> ⅓ cup raw pumpkin seeds
> ⅓ cup pine nuts
> ½ teaspoon salt
> 1 teaspoon chili powder
> 1 egg, beaten
> four 4-ounce trout fillets
> 1 tablespoon olive oil

Place the pumpkin seeds, pine nuts, salt, and chili powder in a food processor and pulse until finely chopped. Transfer the mixture to a plate. Brush the beaten egg on the fish. Dip the flesh side of the fish into the nut mixture.

Heat the olive oil in a nonstick frying pan over medium heat. Add the fish and cook for 3 to 4 minutes, flesh-side down. Flip the fish over, skin-side down, and cook for 4 more minutes. Fish should flake easily with a fork.

Makes 4 servings.

NUTRITION INFORMATION PER SERVING
Calories: 291
Protein: 29 grams
Carbohydrate: 5 grams
Dietary Fiber: 1 gram
Fat: 17 grams
Saturated Fat: 4 grams
Monounsaturated Fat: 7 grams
Polyunsaturated Fat: 5 grams
Cholesterol: 129 milligrams
Sodium: 383 milligrams
Glycemic Index: low

Curried Chickpea Stew with Spinach

Prep Time: 20 minutes

This is a flavorful, easy-to-prepare soup that provides a generous amount of beneficial fiber.

> 1 tablespoon olive oil
> 1 onion, peeled and chopped
> 15-ounce can (1½ cups cooked) chickpeas, rinsed
> 1 cup trimmed fresh spinach
> 2 teaspoons curry powder
> 1 teaspoon freshly ground pepper
> 1 cup water
> 4 ounces baked tofu, cut into small pieces

NUTRITION INFORMATION PER SERVING
Calories: 266
Protein: 15 grams
Carbohydrate: 33 grams
Dietary Fiber: 11 grams
Fat: 10 grams
Saturated Fat: 1 gram
Monounsaturated Fat: 2.2 grams
Polyunsaturated Fat: 0.5 gram
Cholesterol: 0 milligram
Sodium: 688 milligrams
Glycemic Index: low

Heat the oil in a soup pot. Sauté the onion and garlic in the oil for a few minutes. Add the chickpeas, spinach, curry powder, pepper, and water. Cook together, stirring as spinach wilts, for about 5 minutes. Take 1 cup of the pot contents and purée in the blender to thicken. Add back to the pot. Add the tofu pieces and cook for a few more minutes.

Makes 3 servings. Serving size: 1 cup.

Teriyaki Swordfish with Sugar Snap Peas and Portobello Mushrooms

Prep Time: 10 minutes
Cook Time: 10 minutes

This is a simple and flavorful dish. You may substitute white wine for the mirin. Have the fish cut into thinner half-inch pieces, or cut a thick piece in half butterfly fashion to make a thinner steak. Thinner fish cooks faster and cooks more consistently. The wasabi paste gives it some extra heat, so serve it if you like foods with extra spice.

NUTRITION INFORMATION PER SERVING
Calories: 305
Protein: 35 grams
Carbohydrate: 14 grams
Dietary Fiber: 3 grams
Fat: 8 grams
Saturated Fat: 2 grams
Monounsaturated Fat: 2.5 grams
Polyunsaturated Fat: 1.5 grams
Cholesterol: 62 milligrams
Sodium: 423 milligrams
Glycemic Index: low

    12 ounces sugar snap peas
    ¼ cup water
    1 teaspoon fresh grated ginger or ½ teaspoon dried ginger
    2 tablespoons low-sodium soy sauce
    ½ tablespoon toasted sesame oil or peanut oil
    3 tablespoons mirin (Japanese sweetened rice wine)
    1 teaspoon brown sugar
    1 pound swordfish steaks cut ½ inch thick
    8 ounces portobello mushrooms, stems removed, caps sliced ½ inch thick
    1 teaspoon wasabi paste, optional

In a frying pan, cook the sugar snap peas in the water for 2 minutes. Remove from the heat. Combine the ginger, soy sauce, sesame or peanut oil, mirin, and brown sugar in a nonstick fry pan or griddle. Heat the pan over medium heat, then place the fish in the pan and

Teriyaki Swordfish with Sugar Snap Peas (continued)

cook for 1½ minutes on each side. Remove fish from the pan. Using the same pan, cook the mushrooms for 2 minutes, then add the sugar snap peas to the pan juices that remain from cooking the fish and mushrooms.

Serve each piece of fish in the center of each of four dinner plates. Spoon the vegetables around each piece of fish. Mix the wasabi with the water and stir until a paste is formed.

Serve with a teaspoon of wasabi paste on each piece of fish.

Wasabi Paste (optional)

> 1 tablespoon wasabi powder (Japanese horseradish powder)
> 1 tablespoon water

Makes 4 servings.

Spinach Strawberry Salad with Goat Cheese and Chicken
Prep Time: 20 minutes

I love this salad. The fresh spinach and mixed greens offer carotenoids, folate, magnesium, riboflavin, and vitamin B6. The delicious dressing, rich in essential fats, enhances the availability of the fat-soluble carotenoids. The walnuts contain heart-healthy omega-3 fats (alpha-linolenic acid) and protective sterols that help prevent cholesterol from being absorbed into the bloodstream. Strawberries add vitamin C, fiber, and fantastic flavor. Goat cheese, or chèvre, adds a pungent flavor and counters the sweetness of the strawberries just perfectly. To make it more of a main course, top each serving with sliced grilled chicken or salmon.

NUTRITION INFORMATION PER SERVING

Calories: 340
Protein: 24 grams
Carbohydrate: 25 grams
Dietary Fiber: 5 grams
Fat: 17 grams
Saturated Fat: 4 grams
Monounsaturated Fat: 5 grams
Polyunsaturated Fat: 7 grams
Cholesterol: 55 milligrams
Sodium: 266 milligrams
Glycemic Index: low

Chicken

1 bouillon cube in 1 quart water
¾ pound skinless, boneless chicken breasts

Honey-Dijon Dressing

1 tablespoon olive oil
1 tablespoon flaxseed oil
2 tablespoons honey
1 tablespoon orange juice
1 tablespoon lime juice
1 tablespoon rice wine vinegar
2 teaspoons Dijon mustard

Salad

6 cups fresh spinach
2 cups mixed greens
1 cup strawberries, stems removed and sliced
2 kiwi fruit, peeled and cut lengthwise into ¼-inch
   wedges
¼ cup walnuts, chopped
½ cup goat cheese, crumbled (from a plain log or feta)

Bring 1 quart of water and a bouillon cube to a boil in a frying pan; stir to dissolve the cube. Turn heat down to the lowest setting possible and wait for the water to stop boiling. Pound the chicken pieces to ½ inch thick using a mallet. Add the chicken pieces to this liquid and poach for about 6 minutes, until the chicken is cooked. Remove chicken from the pan and slice into bite-size pieces. Set aside.

Prepare Honey-Dijon Dressing by shaking all the dressing ingredients together in a tightly covered jar or blending in a blender. Shake again before pouring over the salad.

Put the greens in a large salad bowl. Add the strawberries, kiwi, and walnuts to the bowl, pour the dressing over the ingredients, and toss the salad to coat with dressing. Add in goat cheese and chicken and toss again.

Makes 4 servings.

Sunflower Burgers

Prep Time: 20 minutes
Cook Time: 10 minutes

These veggie burgers have a nice flavor and can be topped with your choice of cheese. Serve with a plate of your favorite sautéed vegetables.

½ cup textured vegetable protein
½ cup boiling water
1 cup sunflower seeds
1 cup cooked brown rice
½ cup grated carrots
3 eggs
½ teaspoon salt
1 teaspoon black pepper
½ teaspoon chili powder
up to 1 tablespoon canola, peanut, safflower, or corn oil
7 slices low-fat cheese, optional

NUTRITION INFORMATION PER SERVING (WITH CHEESE)
Calories: 306
Protein: 21 grams
Carbohydrate: 17 grams
Dietary Fiber: 5 grams
Fat: 18.6 grams
Saturated Fat: 3 grams
Monounsaturated Fat: 3 grams
Polyunsaturated Fat: 1 gram
Cholesterol: 110 milligrams
Sodium: 513 milligrams
Glycemic Index: low

Combine the textured vegetable protein and boiling water in a measuring cup. Let sit about 15 minutes to increase volume. Grind the sunflower seeds in a food processor for about 45 seconds. Add the soaked textured vegetable protein, brown rice, carrots, eggs, salt, pepper, and chili powder to the food processor and purée until combined.

Make 7 patties out of the sunflower seed mixture. Heat the oil in a nonstick skillet over medium heat. Brown patties for 3 minutes on each side in the heated skillet. If you want cheese on top, add the cheese during the last minute of cooking and cook until it melts.

Makes 7 servings.

Grilled Catfish with Tomato Cilantro Sauce

Prep and Cook Time: 30 minutes

Instead of grilling, this fish can be pan-fried in a nonstick skillet. Other fish varieties that work well with this sauce are fresh tuna, shark, Chilean sea bass, and sea trout.

Nonstick cooking spray
1¼ pounds catfish fillets
juice of 3 limes
1 tablespoon olive oil
1 large garlic clove, peeled and minced
1 small onion, peeled and chopped
½ red bell pepper, chopped
1 cup fresh cilantro (coriander) leaves, chopped
8 plum tomatoes, chopped
½ teaspoon salt

NUTRITION INFORMATION PER SERVING

Calories: 271
Protein: 24 grams
Carbohydrate: 12 grams
Dietary Fiber: 2.4 grams
Fat: 15 grams
Saturated Fat: 3 grams
Monounsaturated Fat: 0.8 gram
Polyunsaturated Fat: 2.8 grams
Cholesterol: 67 milligrams
Sodium: 380 milligrams
Glycemic Index: low

Spray the grill with nonstick cooking spray, then heat. Place catfish fillets on a plate and squeeze juice of 1 lime over top. Set aside.

Make the sauce: Heat the olive oil in a skillet. Add the garlic and onion and sauté for 3 minutes. Add the red bell pepper and sauté for 5 minutes. Add the cilantro, tomatoes, juice of two limes, and salt. Mix, cover, and simmer on low for 10 minutes, stirring often. As the sauce simmers, grill fish for about 5 minutes per side. Check with fork to see if cooked; the flesh will separate easily. Do not overcook.

Place fillets on a large serving platter. Spoon sauce over top and garnish with a little fresh chopped cilantro.

Makes 4 servings.

Turkey Tostadas

Prep Time: 15 minutes
Cook Time: 15 minutes

These are filling and flavorful. Kids love them, too!

2 garlic cloves, peeled and chopped fine
1 small onion, peeled and chopped fine
1 small green pepper, seeded and chopped fine
1 pound ground turkey
1½ tablespoons chili powder
2–3 tablespoons tomato paste
4 tablespoons water
8 corn tortillas

Topping

2 cups shredded lettuce
1 tomato, chopped fine
½ cup low-fat sour cream
½ cup grated cheddar cheese
4 tablespoons fresh chopped cilantro

NUTRITION INFORMATION PER SERVING

Calories: 355
Protein: 31 grams
Carbohydrate: 26 grams
Dietary Fiber: 4.4 grams
Fat: 15 grams
Saturated Fat: 7 grams
Monounsaturated Fat: 0.3 gram
Polyunsaturated Fat: 0.5 gram
Cholesterol: 90 milligrams
Sodium: 261 milligrams
Glycemic Index: low

Preheat oven to 350 degrees. Sauté the garlic, onion, and green pepper for 2 minutes in a nonstick frying pan over medium heat. Add ground turkey, chili powder, tomato paste, and water; continue cooking about 10 minutes until meat is cooked. Stir the meat often to break it up and combine flavors. While the meat is cooking, lay the corn tortillas on a cookie sheet. Bake for 5 minutes.

To assemble each serving: Place 2 corn tortillas on four dinner plates, top with turkey mixture, lettuce, tomato, sour cream, cheddar cheese, and a pinch of cilantro.

Make 4 generous servings. Serving size 2 tostadas.

Picadillo

Prep Time: 15 minutes
Cook Time: 15 minutes

This is a dish of Cuban and South American origin. It is often served with rice or stuffed in dough for empañadas. It is traditionally made with beef, but ground turkey makes it lower in fat and calories.

1 tablespoon olive oil
2–3 garlic cloves, peeled and chopped
1 medium onion, peeled and finely chopped
1 teaspoon cumin powder
½ red bell pepper, seeded and finely chopped
2 small hot chili peppers, seeded and finely chopped
1 pound ground turkey
⅓ cup white wine
3 tablespoons tomato paste
½ cup water
15 green olives stuffed with pimientos, chopped
1–2 tablespoons capers
¼ cup raisins
1 teaspoon cinnamon
½ teaspoon salt (optional)

NUTRITION INFORMATION PER SERVING

Calories: 296
Protein: 24 grams
Carbohydrate: 18 grams
Dietary Fiber: 2.6 grams
Fat: 13 grams
Saturated Fat: 2.5 grams
Monounsaturated Fat: 1.7 grams
Polyunsaturated Fat: 1.6 grams
Cholesterol: 65 milligrams
Sodium: 132 milligrams
Glycemic Index: low

Heat the oil, garlic, and onion in a frying pan. Add the cumin, red bell pepper, chili peppers, and ground turkey. Cook together for about 3 minutes over medium heat, stirring regularly. Add the remaining ingredients and cook together another 5 to 10 minutes, stirring regularly.

Makes 4 servings.

Tilapia with Honey Mustard Sauce

Prep Time: 15 minutes
Cook Time: 15 minutes

2½ tablespoons grainy mustard
1 teaspoon prepared horseradish
1 tablespoon honey
¾ cup plain yogurt
1¼ pounds tilapia
⅓ cup seasoned breadcrumbs
⅓ cup pecans, finely chopped

NUTRITION INFORMATION PER SERVING
Calories: 321
Protein: 34 grams
Carbohydrate: 19 grams
Dietary Fiber: 5 grams
Fat: 12 grams
Saturated Fat: 2 grams
Monounsaturated Fat: 4 grams
Polyunsaturated Fat: 2 grams
Cholesterol: 71 milligrams
Sodium: 478 milligrams
Glycemic Index: low

Preheat oven to 425 degrees. Mix the mustard, horseradish, honey, and yogurt together in a bowl. Transfer ¼ cup of this sauce to a small bowl and set it aside for later. Rinse the fish. Mix the breadcrumbs and chopped pecans on a sheet of foil.

Dip each piece of fish into the yogurt mixture, then dredge the fish in the breadcrumb-pecan mixture to coat lightly. Shake off any extra breading. Lay the coated fish on a foil-lined baking pan. Bake for 10 minutes. Set the oven to broil. Drizzle the sauce you had set aside onto the top of each piece of fish. Broil 3 minutes. Fish should break easily with a fork if it is done.

Makes 4 servings.

Sautéed Peppers and Onions with Turkey Sausage

Prep Time: 10 minutes
Cook Time: 20 minutes

Turkey sausage can be lean or fatty depending on whether the skin and trimmings have been added. Ask how it was made at your local butcher or market.

1 tablespoon canola, peanut, safflower, or corn oil
3 medium onions, peeled and sliced
2 green peppers, seeded and cut into strips
1 red bell pepper, seeded and cut into strips
3-4 garlic cloves, peeled and chopped
1 pound turkey sausage (spicy, sweet, or Italian)
¼ teaspoon salt
fresh ground pepper to taste

NUTRITION INFORMATION PER SERVING

Calories: 299
Protein: 21 grams
Carbohydrate: 20 grams
Dietary Fiber: 4.4 grams
Fat: 16 grams
Saturated Fat: 4.6 grams
Monounsaturated Fat: 2.7 grams
Polyunsaturated Fat: 0.5 gram
Cholesterol: 68 milligrams
Sodium: 880 milligrams
Glycemic Index: low

Heat oil in a skillet; add the onions, green and red peppers, and garlic and cook, stirring often, until onions are soft. Add the turkey sausage; continue cooking, turning sausage occasionally until it is cooked. Add the salt and pepper.

Makes 4 servings

Salmon in BBQ Sauce with Waldorf Salad

Prep Time: 20 minutes
Cook Time: 10 minutes

3 medium apples
½ cup chopped celery
⅛ cup chopped walnuts
¼ cup light mayonnaise
½ cup barbecue sauce
1 pound fresh salmon fillet cut into 4 4-ounce pieces
1½ tablespoons olive oil
2 tablespoons balsamic vinegar
1 teaspoon prepared mustard
fresh ground pepper
pinch of salt
6 cups lettuce leaves

NUTRITION
INFORMATION PER
SERVING
Calories: 414
Protein: 32 grams
Carbohydrate: 21 grams
Dietary Fiber: 5.3 grams
Fat: 23 grams
Saturated Fat: 3.3 grams
Monounsaturated Fat:
  7.5 grams
Polyunsaturated Fat: 6.1
  grams
Cholesterol: 86
  milligrams
Sodium: 367 milligrams
Glycemic Index: low

Core the apples. Chop into ½-inch cubes. Mix them in a bowl with the celery, walnuts, and mayonnaise. Set aside.

Heat the barbecue sauce over medium heat in a nonstick frying pan. Add the salmon fillets and cook for about 4 to 5 minutes on each side. Salmon should easily separate when cut with a fork.

Make a dressing with the olive oil, balsamic vinegar, mustard, pepper, and salt.

Mix the lettuce with the dressing.

Place 1½ cups of the dressed lettuce on each of four dinner plates. Place a piece of salmon on each plate. Place the apple mixture on top of the dressed lettuce.

Makes 4 servings.

Vegetarian Chili

Prep Time: 15 minutes
Cook Time: 25 minutes

Textured vegetable protein is a dry, crumbly soy product that is rich in protein. It is available in health food stores. If soaked in hot water, it expands in volume. In this recipe the textured vegetable protein is added to the hot chili and it absorbs the flavorful sauce. Use the smaller amount of chili powder if you like it milder!

NUTRITION INFORMATION PER SERVING
Calories: 312
Protein: 21 grams
Carbohydrate: 46 grams
Dietary Fiber: 14 grams
Fat: 6 grams
Saturated Fat: 3 grams
Monounsaturated Fat: 1.4 grams
Polyunsaturated Fat: 0.4 gram
Cholesterol: 13 milligrams
Sodium: 530 milligrams
Glycemic Index: low

1 tablespoon canola, peanut, safflower, or corn oil
3 garlic cloves, peeled and chopped
1 medium onion, peeled and chopped
1 medium green pepper, seeded and chopped
1 medium red pepper, seeded and chopped
1–2 tablespoons chili powder
1 teaspoon oregano
2 teaspoons ground cumin
two 28-ounce cans crushed tomatoes
two 15-ounce cans pinto or kidney beans, rinsed
1 cup canned corn, drained
1 cup textured vegetable protein
1 teaspoon salt

Garnishes

½ cup grated cheddar cheese
½ cup low-fat sour cream
½ cup chopped cilantro (coriander)

In a large, heavy-gauge pot, heat the oil and sauté the garlic, onion, green and red peppers for 5 minutes. Add the chili powder, oregano, cumin, tomatoes, and beans. Cook for 15 minutes. Add the corn, textured vegetable protein, and salt and heat through. Garnish each serving with cheese, sour cream, and cilantro.

Makes 8 servings.

Chicken Cacciatore

Prep Time: 20 minutes
Cook Time: 25 minutes

1 tablespoon olive oil
2–3 garlic cloves, peeled and chopped
1 onion, peeled and chopped
1 pound boneless and skinless chicken breasts
½ green bell pepper, seeded and sliced
½ red bell pepper, seeded and sliced
8 ounces mushrooms, halved
1 pound fresh tomatoes, chopped
1 teaspoon fresh thyme
2 teaspoons fresh rosemary
¼ cup fresh chopped basil
½ teaspoon salt
fresh ground pepper to taste
high-protein pasta, optional according to your plan,
   women's or men's; ½ cup each serving

NUTRITION INFORMATION PER SERVING (WITHOUT PASTA)
Calories: 154
Protein: 46 grams
Carbohydrate: 15 grams
Dietary Fiber: 0.5 gram
Fat: 5 grams
Saturated Fat: 0.8 gram
Monounsaturated Fat: 0.8 gram
Polyunsaturated Fat: 0.7 gram
Cholesterol: 27 milligrams
Sodium: 323 milligrams
Glycemic Index: low

Heat the oil in a frying pan. Sauté the garlic and onion in the oil. Sear the chicken on each side for 2 minutes. Remove the chicken and set aside.

Add the green and red peppers, mushrooms, tomatoes, thyme, rosemary, and basil to the onions and garlic; cook together for 5 minutes. Season the vegetables with salt and pepper.

Return the chicken to the pan and cook on each side for 5 minutes over low heat. Remove from the sauce, and slice meat on the diagonal. Return the meat to the sauce and cook 1 more minute.

Serve over high-protein pasta or by itself.

Makes 4 servings.

Mussels Marinara

Prep Time: 20 minutes
Cook Time: 25 minutes

This is a wonderful dish served along with a salad or over a small serving of lower-glycemic pasta.

3 garlic cloves, peeled and chopped
1 medium onion, peeled and chopped
2 bay leaves
1 tablespoon olive oil
28-ounce can crushed tomatoes
¼ cup fresh basil leaves, or 1 tablespoon dried basil
2 teaspoons fresh thyme, or 1 teaspoon dried thyme
1 teaspoon crushed red pepper
2 pounds fresh mussels

NUTRITION INFORMATION PER SERVING

Calories: 294
Protein: 31 grams
Carbohydrate: 24 grams
Dietary Fiber: 4 grams
Fat: 9 grams
Saturated Fat: 1.5 grams
Monounsaturated Fat: 3.9 grams
Polyunsaturated Fat: 1.7 grams
Cholesterol: 64 milligrams
Sodium: 224 milligrams
Glycemic Index: low

In a heavy pot, sauté the garlic, onions, and bay leaves in the olive oil for 3 minutes. Add the crushed tomatoes, basil, thyme, and red pepper and let sauce simmer on low for 10 minutes while you prepare the mussels.

Put the mussels in a bowl of cold water and rinse until the water is clean and free of sand. Do this carefully, as the taste of sand in your food will stop you from eating mussels again in the near future. There is often a small, black hairy clump in the outside of the shell called the beard. As you sort through the mussels, pull this off if you find it. (The beard is what the mussel uses to attach to rocks or shells in the water.) Discard any mussels that are open before cooking. Fresh live mussels will stay tightly closed and will open only upon steaming. Any mussels that don't open after 5 minutes should also be discarded.

Once the mussels are clean and debearded, add them to the hot pot of sauce. Cover and cook over medium-low heat for 5 to 7 minutes, stirring once or twice. The mussels should open during this steaming.

Makes 4 servings.

Shrimp in Thai Red Curry Sauce

Prep Time: 30 minutes
Cook Time: 10 minutes

Spicy and delicious! Serve this with brown rice.

1 tablespoon toasted sesame, peanut, or canola oil
2 garlic cloves, peeled and chopped
2 thin slices ginger, peeled and chopped
2 tablespoons finely chopped fresh lemongrass
1 tablespoon Thai Red Curry Paste (available at Asian and health food stores)
1¼ pounds shrimp, peeled and deveined
8 medium mushrooms, quartered with stems trimmed
1 red bell pepper, seeded and cut into strips
1 medium zucchini, cut into pieces
½ cup coconut milk
1 tablespoon fresh lime juice
1 tablespoon Thai fish sauce (available at Asian stores)
¼ cup fresh chopped basil

NUTRITION INFORMATION PER SERVING

Calories: 211
Protein: 20 grams
Carbohydrate: 6.8 grams
Dietary Fiber: 1.7 grams
Fat: 12 grams
Saturated Fat: 6.5 grams
Monounsaturated Fat: 0.4 gram
Polyunsaturated Fat: 0.5 gram
Cholesterol: 168 milligrams
Sodium: 742 milligrams
Glycemic Index: low

Heat the oil, garlic, ginger, and lemongrass in a wok or large frying pan over medium heat for 2 minutes. Add the curry paste and the shrimp and stir-fry for 2 minutes, stirring often. Make sure the curry paste thins and breaks down. Add the mushrooms, red bell pepper, and zucchini and cook for 2 more minutes. Add the remaining ingredients and cook for 2 more minutes.

Makes 4 servings.

Cheese Ravioli with Tomato Basil Sauce

Prep Time: 15 minutes
Cook Time: 30 minutes

2 teaspoons canola, peanut, safflower, or corn oil
3 garlic cloves, peeled and chopped
1 medium onion, peeled and chopped
2 pounds fresh tomatoes, cored and chopped, or
    28-ounce can Italian plum tomatoes
1 pound cheese- or spinach-cheese-filled ravioli
½ cup fresh basil
½ teaspoon salt
fresh ground pepper or crushed red pepper to taste
3 cups fresh broccoli florets
4 tablespoons Parmesan cheese

NUTRITION INFORMATION PER SERVING
Calories: 393
Protein: 18.5 grams
Carbohydrate: 53 grams
Dietary Fiber: 7 grams
Fat: 13 grams
Saturated Fat: 5 grams
Monounsaturated Fat: 4.4 grams
Polyunsaturated Fat: 0.7 gram
Cholesterol: 49 milligrams
Sodium: 596 milligrams
Glycemic Index: low

Heat the oil, garlic, and onion together in a pot over low heat for a few minutes to lightly brown. Add the tomatoes and cook for 10 minutes over low heat, covered.

Bring 2 quarts of water to a boil in a pot large enough for the ravioli. Add the ravioli and cook according to package instructions. Drain when cooked and set aside.

Add the basil and salt to the purée. Purée the sauce in batches in the blender. (Use caution when puréeing hot liquids.) Return to the pot. Season with pepper. Add the broccoli to the sauce and cook for 5 minutes on low heat. Mix the cooked ravioli, sauce, and broccoli together in a bowl. Top each serving with a tablespoon of Parmesan cheese.

Makes 4 servings.

Black Bean Stew

Prep Time: 20 minutes
Cook Time: 25 minutes (using canned beans)

This stew is hearty, healthy, and filling. It can be made with turkey sausage, bits of turkey ham, or turkey bacon. If you'd like to make it completely vegetarian, you can add textured vegetable protein soaked in hot water.

NUTRITION INFORMATION PER SERVING

Calories: 319
Protein: 22 grams
Carbohydrate: 41 grams
Dietary Fiber: 11 grams
Fat: 9 grams
Saturated Fat: 3 grams
Monounsaturated Fat: 0.6 gram
Polyunsaturated Fat: 0.2 gram
Cholesterol: 39 milligrams
Sodium: 609 milligrams
Glycemic Index: low

1½ cups dried black beans, cooked according to directions below, or three 15-ounce cans black beans, rinsed

1 teaspoon olive oil

1 medium onion, peeled and chopped

2–3 garlic cloves, peeled and chopped

2 teaspoons ground cumin seed

1 whole jalapeño pepper, seeded

2 yellow, red, or orange bell peppers, seeded and chopped

¾ pound lean turkey sausage, vegetarian-based sausage, or 1 cup textured vegetable protein soaked in 1 cup boiled water

6–8 plum tomatoes, chopped, or 2 cups Italian plum tomatoes

juice of 2 limes

1 cup bean broth or water

1 teaspoon salt (omit if using canned beans)

¾ cup chopped cilantro (coriander)

6 tablespoons chopped scallions

6 tablespoons low-fat sour cream

If using dried beans, soak and cook according to directions below. Heat the oil in a soup pot, then add the onion, garlic, cumin, jalapeño and bell peppers. Cook for 5 minutes over low heat. Add the turkey or vegetarian sausage and continue cooking for about 10 minutes over low heat. (If using textured vegetable protein, add it during the next step.) Add the cooked beans, tomatoes, lime juice, broth or water, salt, and cilantro. Cook together for 5 minutes.

Remove whole jalapeño before serving. Top with a sprinkle of scallions and sour cream.

Makes 6 servings. Serving size: 1½ cups.

To cook black beans: Pick through the beans to eliminate any dirt and small stones. Put the beans in a pot and add 6 cups water. Bring the beans to a boil for a minute, then turn the heat off and let the beans sit for an hour. They will swell while soaking. After an hour, discard the soaking water. Fill the pot with one cup of cooking liquid, and simmer the beans for a 30 minutes. They should be tender at this point.

Spinach Mushroom Crepes

Prep Time: 30 minutes
Cook Time: 15 minutes

These are really good and very satisfying.

Crepes (Makes four 8-inch crepes)

⅓ cup whole-wheat flour
3 tablespoons gluten flour
½ teaspoon baking powder
⅛ teaspoon salt
1 teaspoon melted butter
1 egg
⅓ cup skim milk
⅓ cup water

Filling

½ pound mushrooms
10 ounces fresh spinach, stems trimmed

Sauce

1 tablespoon butter
1½ tablespoons white unbleached flour
1 cup skim milk
3 ounces Swiss cheese, grated (about ⅔ cup packed)
¼ teaspoon salt
⅛ teaspoon ground white pepper

NUTRITION INFORMATION PER SERVING
Calories: 275
Protein: 17 grams
Carbohydrate: 28 grams
Dietary Fiber: 5 grams
Fat: 12 grams
Saturated Fat: 8 grams
Monounsaturated Fat: 0.1 gram
Polyunsaturated Fat: 0.2 gram
Cholesterol: 95 milligrams
Sodium: 433 milligrams
Glycemic Index: low

Spinach Mushroom Crepes (continued)

To make the crepes: Mix together all the dry crepe ingredients in a bowl, then add the wet ingredients. Whisk until lump-free. Lightly oil or butter a well-seasoned 8-inch crepe pan or nonstick crepe pan. Heat over medium-low heat, then pour ¼ cup of the batter in the pan, gently tip the pan all around to spread the batter, and quickly pour back any excess batter. Heat over low heat until crepe cooks. The appearance will change from moist to dry. Flip carefully using a spatula and cook for 30 seconds on the other side. Transfer to a plate, then repeat the process for the remaining 3 crepes.

Set aside until needed.

To make the filling: Sauté the mushrooms and spinach in a pot over medium-low heat for a few minutes until the spinach wilts. Drain off excess liquid. Set aside.

To make the sauce: Heat the butter in a saucepan over low heat. Whisk in the flour, stirring to mix flour into melted butter. It will look pasty. Slowly add the milk, stirring as the mixture thickens, then add the grated cheese. The sauce will continue to thicken. Season the sauce with salt and pepper. Remove from heat.

To put together: Preheat oven to 400 degrees. Mix ½ cup of the sauce into the filling.

Place about ½ cup of the vegetable mixture in the middle of each crepe. Spread the filling out lengthwise, then roll the crepe over the filling and over again into a cylinder shape. Place on a lightly oiled pan. Repeat with the remaining filling and crepes. Bake uncovered for 5 minutes. Top with the remaining sauce and bake for 5 more minutes.

Makes 4 crepes. Serving size: 1 crepe.

Southwestern Meatloaf

Prep Time: 10 minutes
Cook Time: 40 minutes

This meatloaf has a slightly spicy twist.

½ onion, peeled and finely chopped
2 garlic cloves, peeled and chopped
1½ pounds lean ground beef, preferably 90% lean
¼ cup barbecue sauce
1 egg
½ teaspoon salt
1 tablespoon chili powder

Preheat oven to 350 degrees. Mix all ingredients together
in a bowl. Shape into a loaf and transfer to a loaf pan.
    Bake for 40 minutes.

Makes 4 servings.

NUTRITION
INFORMATION PER
SERVING
Calories: 257
Protein: 35 grams
Carbohydrate: 10 grams
Dietary Fiber: 1 gram
Fat: 9 grams
Saturated Fat: 3 grams
Monounsaturated Fat:
    3.6 grams
Polyunsaturated Fat: 1.1
    grams
Cholesterol: 152
    milligrams
Sodium: 617 milligrams
Glycemic Index: low

Teriyaki Beef and Broccoli

Prep Time and Cook Time: 30 minutes
Marinating Time: 30 minutes (or overnight)

Marinate the beef overnight and cook brown rice in
advance so that this delicious recipe can be ready with
just a few minutes of last minute stir-frying.

¾ pound lean sirloin steak, boneless
2 teaspoons tamari soy sauce
2 teaspoons sesame oil
¼ cup homemade low-fat chicken or beef broth, or
    canned low-fat and low-sodium
1 tablespoon sherry
1 teaspoon minced garlic
1 teaspoon finely chopped ginger root
1 pound broccoli florets
1 tablespoon peanut oil
1 teaspoon cornstarch
2 tablespoons cold water
2 cups cooked brown rice

NUTRITION
INFORMATION PER
SERVING
Calories: 338
Protein: 24 grams
Carbohydrate: 30 grams
Dietary Fiber: 5 grams
Fat: 14 grams
Saturated Fat: 4 grams
Monounsaturated Fat: 5
    grams
Polyunsaturated Fat: 2
    grams
Cholesterol: 49
    milligrams
Sodium: 305 milligrams
Glycemic Index: low

Teriyaki Beef and Broccoli (ocntinued)

Cut the beef into thin diagonal strips. Mix the tamari, sesame oil, chicken or beef broth, sherry, garlic, and ginger in a bowl large enough to also hold the meat. Marinate the beef in this mixture for 30 minutes or overnight.

Place the broccoli in a microwave safe bowl and cover. Microwave on high for 3 minutes.

Heat the peanut oil in a wok or large frying pan over medium heat. Add the beef and half of the marinade and stir-fry for 2 minutes until brown. Remove the beef from the pan and set aside. Add the broccoli and remaining marinade and stir-fry for 5 minutes, adding a little more stock if necessary.

Stir the cornstarch in the 2 tablespoons of cold water until dissolved. Add to the pan along with the beef; cook another minute so that the cornstarch thickens the sauce. Serve over the brown rice.

Makes 4 servings.

Grilled Ratatouille with Shrimp or Tofu

Prep Time: 40 minutes
Cook Time: 20 minutes

Ratatouille is a dish from Provence that combines a variety of vegetables, garlic and herbs, marinated in olive oil. Add your choice of shrimp or tofu.

> 1 pound medium shrimp, peeled and deveined, or
>   1 pound extra-firm tofu cut into 1-inch cubes
> 1 small eggplant (about ¾ pound)
> ¾ teaspoon sea salt
> ½ pound zucchini (2 small)
> 1 medium green bell pepper
> 1 small onion, peeled

NUTRITION INFORMATION PER SERVING: (WITH SHRIMP)

Calories: 189
Protein: 18 grams
Carbohydrate: 15 grams
Dietary Fiber: 3.6 grams
Fat: 7 grams
Saturated Fat: 1 gram
Monounsaturated Fat: 3.8 grams
Polyunsaturated Fat: 1 gram
Cholesterol: 115 milligrams
Sodium: 765 milligrams
Glycemic Index: low

Dressing

2 tablespoons olive oil
¼ cup rice vinegar
2 tablespoons water
½ teaspoon sea salt
1 tablespoon chopped fresh basil
1 garlic clove, peeled and minced

1 cup low-fat spaghetti sauce, heated

NUTRITION
INFORMATION
PER SERVING
(WITH TOFU)
Calories: 182
Protein: 10 grams
Carbohydrate: 16 grams
Dietary Fiber: 4 grams
Fat: 10 grams
Saturated Fat: 1.4 grams
Monounsaturated Fat:
    4.6 grams
Polyunsaturated Fat: 3.2
    grams
Cholesterol: 0 milligram
Sodium: 660 milligrams
Glycemic Index: low

Rinse the shrimp and set aside. Cut the eggplant into 1-inch chunks. Place the eggplant in a colander over a bowl or sink. Sprinkle with the sea salt and let drain for 30 minutes. Rinse and pat dry. Spray grill with nonstick cooking spray. Preheat grill.

Cut the zucchini, pepper, and onion into 1-inch chunks. Thread the shrimp (or tofu), eggplant, zucchini, pepper, and onion alternately on each of six 10-inch metal skewers, leaving a little space between each item. (*Note:* If you use wooden skewers, be sure to soak them in water prior to threading on the food.)

Prepare the dressing by blending or shaking the olive oil, vinegar, water, sea salt, basil, and garlic together. Brush kabobs with the dressing.

Grill the kabobs 4 to 6 inches from medium heat for 15 to 20 minutes with the grill top down, turning and brushing twice with the dressing. The vegetables should be crisp-tender and the shrimp (or tofu) cooked throughout.

Heat the spaghetti sauce in a small pan while the kabobs are grilling, stirring occasionally. Serve the kabobs with the pasta sauce.

Makes 6 servings.

Eggplant Parmesan

Prep Time: 15 minutes
Cook Time: 1 hour

Instead of frying the eggplant, bake it! Wheat germ is a great breading product and has essential fats and protein, too.

NUTRITION
INFORMATION PER
SERVING
Calories: 220
Protein: 18 grams
Carbohydrate: 17 grams
Dietary Fiber: 5 grams
Fat: 10 grams
Saturated Fat: 5 grams
Monounsaturated Fat: 3
grams
Polyunsaturated Fat: 1.3
grams
Cholesterol: 53
milligrams
Sodium: 332 milligrams
Glycemic Index: low

2 medium eggplants

2 eggs

½ cup milk

½ teaspoon salt

1 cup toasted wheat germ

1½ cups spaghetti sauce (or use Tomato Basil Sauce, page 209)

2 cups grated part-skim mozzarella cheese

½ cup grated Parmesan cheese

½ cup fresh chopped basil leaves

1 tsp. olive oil (optional)

Peel the eggplant with a vegetable peeler or a small serrated paring knife. Cut width-wise into ½-inch slices. Preheat oven to 350 degrees. Mix the eggs, milk, and salt in a bowl. Pour the wheat germ on a plate or a piece of foil. Dip each piece of eggplant into the egg mixture, then into the wheat germ, coating the eggplant on both sides. Lay coated eggplant pieces on lightly oiled baking pans or pans lined with parchment paper and bake for 20 minutes.

Coat the bottom of a 9-by-12-inch pan with ¾ cup spaghetti sauce. Place half of the baked eggplant on the bottom. Top with half of the cheeses and half of the basil. Repeat layering with the remaining eggplant, sauce, cheeses, and basil. Cover with foil and bake for 30 minutes. Remove foil and bake for 5 more minutes.

Makes 8 servings.

Marinated Asian Beef Salad

Prep Time: 30 minutes
Marinating Time: 30 minutes
Cook Time: 10 minutes

This is a delicious salad. Enjoy!

Marinade

1 tablespoon low-sodium soy sauce

2 garlic cloves, peeled and chopped

2 tablespoon white wine

3 tablespoons lime juice

1 pound flank steak

nonstick cooking spray

Dressing

1 teaspoon grated ginger

¼ cup chopped cilantro (coriander) or basil

2 garlic cloves, peeled and chopped

1 tablespoon honey

1 tablespoon Thai or Vietnamese fish sauce (available at Asian food stores)

¼ cup fresh lime juice

¼ cup fresh lemon juice

1 teaspoon chili powder or 1 tablespoon fresh chopped and seeded green hot chili pepper

Salad

6 ounces fresh baby spinach or 1 head romaine lettuce

1 pound cucumber, cut into bite-size pieces

1 pound tomatoes, cut into chunks

½ cup fresh chopped mint

½ red onion, peeled and sliced into thin strips

NUTRITION INFORMATION PER SERVING

Calories: 291
Protein: 28 grams
Carbohydrate: 26 grams
Dietary Fiber: 5 grams
Fat: 9 grams
Saturated Fat: 4 grams
Monounsaturated Fat: 3.4 grams
Polyunsaturated Fat: 0.4 gram
Cholesterol: 57 milligrams
Sodium: 644 milligrams
Glycemic Index: low

Combine the soy sauce, garlic, wine, and lime juice in a container wide enough to fit the flank steak. Marinate steak in refrigerator for 30 minutes, turning the meat over at least once while marinating.

Combine the dressing ingredients in a bowl or a food processor and blend. Set aside.

Marinated Asian Beef Salad (continued)

Preheat grill and spray with nonstick cooking spray.
Tear the spinach or lettuce into bite-size pieces.
Divide among 4 dinner plates.

Spray grill with nonstick spray and ook the meat on
the grill for 4 to 5 minutes per side. Remove, test for
doneness, then, if done, slice the meat on the diagonal
into thin strips. Mix the meat and the meat juices in a
bowl with the chunks of cucumber, tomato, chopped
mint, red onion, and dressing. Stir to coat. Divide this
mixture onto the top of the four lettuce-dressed plates.

Makes 4 servings.

Turkey London Broil

Prep Time: 5 minutes
Marinating Time: 1 hour
Cook Time: 15 minutes

*This Turkey London Broil is a delicious preparation of
the skinless breast of turkey. Usually it comes in 1½- to
2-pound pieces. It is very lean, and when marinated, is
very flavorful. This recipe is good any time of year and it
is as easy as can be. Serve it with a few vegetables or
corn on the cob or roasted new potatoes (they are lower-
glycemic than baked potatoes).*

Marinade

½ cup orange juice
¼ cup maple syrup
¼ cup ketchup
1 tablespoon chili powder
1 tablespoon low-sodium soy sauce

1 pound turkey London broil
nonstick cooking spray

Combine ingredients for the marinade in a bowl. Place
the turkey London broil in the marinade and marinate
in the refrigerator for 1 hour.

NUTRITION
INFORMATION PER
SERVING

Calories: 211
Protein: 9 grams
Carbohydrate: 21 grams
Dietary Fiber: 0.5 gram
Fat: 1 gram
Saturated Fat: 0.3 gram
Monounsaturated Fat:
  0.2 gram
Polyunsaturated Fat: 0.3
  gram
Cholesterol: 70
  milligrams
Sodium: 375 milligrams
Glycemic Index: low

If grilling: Spray the grill with nonstick cooking spray and preheat. Place the meat on the grill and cook about 5 minutes per side. Drizzle with a little marinade as it cooks. Check to see if the meat is completely cooked. If not, cook another minute or two on each side.

If broiling: Set the broiler rack about 3 inches below the heat source. Line the bottom of a broiler pan with foil; place the marinated meat on the top pan of the broiler pan. Broil about 5 minutes per side. Check to see if the meat is cooked; if not, cook another minute or two on each side.

Makes 4 servings.

Beef Stew

Prep Time: 20 minutes
Cook Time: 60 minutes

Here's an updated version of an old favorite using lower glycemic ingredients.

1 tablespoon olive oil

1 pound lean beef cubes

3 garlic cloves, peeled and chopped

1 onion, peeled and chopped

2 bay leaves

2 teaspoons fresh rosemary or 1 teaspoon dried rosemary

1 teaspoon fresh thyme or ½ teaspoon dried thyme

3 cups chicken or beef broth, preferably unsalted or low-sodium

1 cup red wine

4 medium carrots, peeled and cut into chunks

3 stalks celery, cut into chunks

½ pound new (not Idaho) potatoes, cut into halves or quarters

1 cup fresh or frozen peas

1 cup canned corn, drained

1 tablespoon cornstarch dissolved in ¼ cup cold water

½ teaspoon salt (if using unsalted chicken stock)

½ teaspoon fresh ground pepper

NUTRITION INFORMATION PER SERVING

Calories: 387
Protein: 31 grams
Carbohydrate: 38 grams
Dietary Fiber: 7.6 grams
Fat: 11 grams
Saturated Fat: 3 grams
Monounsaturated Fat: 5.2 grams
Polyunsaturated Fat: 0.8 gram
Cholesterol: 71 milligrams
Sodium: 260 milligrams
Glycemic Index: low

Beef Stew (continued)

Heat the oil in a large, heavy pot. Add the beef cubes, garlic, and onion and cook on medium heat for 5 minutes, stirring to brown the meat on all sides. Add the bay leaves, rosemary, thyme, chicken or beef broth, and wine. Cook for 20 minutes on low heat, covered. Add the carrots, celery, and new potatoes and cook for 20 minutes more on low heat, covered.

In a bowl, mix the cornstarch with the cold water; stir until lump-free. Add to the stew, stirring as the sauce thickens and clears. Add peas and corn and season with salt and pepper. Cook for 10 more minutes over low heat, covered.

Makes 4 servings.

Chicken Kabobs with Dates

Prep Time: 15 minutes
Marinating Time: 1 hour
Cook Time: 6 minutes

The marinade gives the chicken flavor and keeps it moist with dry broiler heat.

Marinade

> juice of 1 lemon
> juice of 1 lime
> 1 tablespoon apple juice concentrate or 3 tablespoons
> unsweetened apple juice
> 1 teaspoon grated lemon peel
> 2 garlic cloves, peeled and minced
> 1 tablespoon low-sodium soy sauce
> ¼ teaspoon fresh ground pepper

Kabobs

> 1 pound boneless and skinless chicken breasts, trimmed
> of excess fat
> 1 medium zucchini, cut into ½-inch chunks

NUTRITION INFORMATION PER SERVING

Calories: 233
Protein: 28 grams
Carbohydrate: 25 grams
Dietary Fiber: 3.3 grams
Fat: 3 grams
Saturated Fat: 0.8 gram
Monounsaturated Fat: 0.9 gram
Polyunsaturated Fat: 0.7 gram
Cholesterol: 67 milligrams
Sodium: 196 milligrams
Glycemic Index: low

1 medium onion, peeled and cut into eighths
½ pound whole mushrooms
1 red bell pepper, seeded and cut into cubes
8 dates, cut in half

Combine the marinade ingredients in a bowl. Cut the chicken into 1-inch cubes. Add the chicken to the marinade, cover with foil or plastic, and refrigerate for at least 1 hour.

Soak 8 bamboo skewers in water or use stainless steel skewers. Arrange the chicken, zucchini, onion, mushrooms, pepper, and dates alternately on the skewers. Set on a pan suitable for the broiler. Broil 3 minutes on each side.

Makes 4 servings. Serving size: 2 skewers.

Shepherd's Pie

Prep Time: 30 minutes
Cook Time: 1 hour

This dish is perfect for a cool day. It can be made ahead. Mashed potatoes make up the crust. The filling is ground turkey and vegetables. If you like the flavor of meat and potatoes, this dish is just right for you.

2¼ pounds red new potatoes (not Idaho), peeled and cut into 2-inch cubes
2 tablespoons butter
¼ cup nonfat milk
¾ teaspoon salt
¼ teaspoon white pepper
1 pound ground turkey
1½ cups frozen mixed vegetables
½ teaspoon fresh ground pepper

NUTRITION INFORMATION PER SERVING
Calories: 415
Protein: 30 grams
Carbohydrate: 43 grams
Dietary Fiber: 6.5 grams
Fat: 13 grams
Saturated Fat: 6 grams
Monounsaturated Fat: 0 gram
Polyunsaturated Fat: 0 gram
Cholesterol: 80 milligrams
Sodium: 603 milligrams
Glycemic Index: low

Cover potatoes with water in a large pot. Simmer for 25 to 30 minutes or until fork tender. Drain off the cooking water. Using a potato masher or ricer, mash the

Shepherd's Pie (continued)

potatoes. Stir in the butter, milk, salt, and pepper. This can be done by hand in a bowl or with an electric mixer.

Preheat oven to 325°.

Line a pie pan with half of the mashed potatoes to form a crust. Using a spoon, push potatoes on the inner edges of the pie pan up to form the edge of the pie crust. Cook the ground turkey in a nonstick frying pan, stirring occasionally. Add the frozen vegetables and pepper. When the meat mixture is cooked, spoon it into the mashed potato–lined pie pan as the filling.

Spread the remaining mashed potatoes around the top outside of the pie.

Bake at 325 degrees for 20 minutes.

Makes 4 servings.

Chicken with Cabbage in Spicy Peanut Dressing

Prep Time: 30 minutes
Cook Time: 1 hour (using whole chicken)

Strips of chicken with an Asian-inspired coleslaw. The flavors combine well to please all of your taste buds.

Dressing

> 2–3 garlic cloves, peeled and chopped
> 2 tablespoons peeled and finely chopped fresh ginger root
> 6 tablespoons peanut butter
> 1 tablespoon white miso or other miso paste*
> 2 hot chili peppers or 1–2 teaspoons chili paste
> 1½ tablespoons rice vinegar
> ⅓ cup water
> 1 teaspoon fructose or granulated sugar
> juice of 2 limes

NUTRITION INFORMATION PER SERVING

Calories: 345
Protein: 34 grams
Carbohydrate: 22 grams
Dietary Fiber: 6 grams
Fat: 15 grams
Saturated Fat: 3 grams
Monounsaturated Fat: 6.6 grams
Polyunsaturated Fat: 4.2 grams
Cholesterol: 67 milligrams
Sodium: 404 milligrams
Glycemic Index: low

Salad

  1 fryer chicken, about 3 pounds, or 1 pound boneless
    breast of chicken
  5 cups grated white cabbage or napa cabbage
  ¾ cup grated fresh carrot (about 3 medium carrots)

Put all the dressing ingredients in the blender or food processor and blend to make the dressing. Set aside.

If using a fryer, simmer chicken in a pot with 2 quarts of water for 1 hour, as if you were making chicken soup. Remove the chicken from the pot and keep the broth as soup stock for another recipe. It will freeze well. Let the chicken cool. Remove the skin and bones and cut the chicken into bite-size strips. Set aside.

If using the boneless chicken breasts, cut them into pieces and marinate them for 1 hour in ¼ cup of the dressing. Sauté the boneless breast of chicken in a non-stick skillet in 1 teaspoon olive oil until cooked.

Mix the cabbage and carrots together, then add the cooked chicken. Mix in the dressing. Let sit 10 minutes, then serve.

Makes 4 servings.

*Miso is a soybean paste. There are many varieties. I like the white or mellow white miso for this dish, though I have used the brown miso, too. Miso is found in health food stores and Asian markets.

Thai Chicken with Broccoli

Prep Time: 20 minutes
Marinating Time: 1–2 hours
Cook Time: 10 minutes

Fish sauce is made from salted, fermented anchovies and adds a very interesting flavor. If you can't find it in the international section at your local grocery store and don't have an Asian food market nearby, use another 1½ tablespoons sodium-reduced soy sauce or tamari.

Marinade

2 tablespoons Thai or Vietnamese fish sauce (nam pla)
½ tablespoon sodium-reduced soy sauce or tamari
1 tablespoon chopped cilantro (coriander)

1 pound boneless and skinless chicken breasts, cut into 1-inch cubes
1 head broccoli, cut into florets
4 medium carrots, peeled and cut into ½-inch pieces
1 tablespoon toasted sesame oil
2 garlic cloves, peeled and finely chopped
2 green Thai fresh chili peppers, chopped (or other hot chili pepper measuring about 1 teaspoon, chopped)
1 tablespoon peeled, chopped ginger root
1 leek, green top and root cut off, white stem split in half to clean, then sliced into quarter-inch slices

NUTRITION INFORMATION PER SERVING

Calories: 230
Protein: 29 grams
Carbohydrate: 15 grams
Dietary Fiber: 3.8 grams
Fat: 6.4 grams
Saturated Fat: 1.3 grams
Monounsaturated Fat: 0.9 gram
Polyunsaturated Fat: 0.7 gram
Cholesterol: 67 milligrams
Sodium: 695 milligrams
Glycemic Index: low

Combine marinade ingredients and marinate chicken cubes for 1 to 2 hours in the refrigerator. Drain the marinade from the chicken, saving both the marinade and the chicken separately.

Place the broccoli and carrots in a microwave-safe bowl with 1 tablespoon of water and cover with plastic wrap. Microwave vegetables for 3 minutes on high (or steam broccoli and carrots in a steamer on top of the stove for about 4 minutes.) Set aside.

Heat the sesame oil in a wok or large frying pan. Add the garlic, chopped chili peppers, ginger, and leek. Sauté for 1 minute. Add the chicken and stir-fry 2 to 3 minutes until the chicken turns from pink to white on all sides. Move the chicken to the sides of the wok. Add the broccoli, carrots, and remaining marinade and stir-fry for 1 minute.

Make 4 servings.

Arroz Con Pollo

Prep Time: 20 minutes
Marinating Time: 1 hour
Cook Time: 1 hour

This is a typical Hispanic dish, full of flavor and very satisfying. It is also very easy to make and great for serving a crowd. If you don't like dark meat, substitute a half-pound of boneless chicken breasts for the thighs and legs.

NUTRITION INFORMATION PER SERVING

Calories: 407
Protein: 37 grams
Carbohydrate: 46 grams
Dietary Fiber: 4.4 grams
Fat: 8 grams
Saturated Fat: 2 grams
Monounsaturated Fat: 3.2 grams
Polyunsaturated Fat: 2 grams
Cholesterol: 96 milligrams
Sodium: 855 milligrams
Glycemic Index: low

1½ pounds boneless and skinless chicken breasts
1 pound chicken thighs and legs
2 teaspoons adobo seasoning (*see recipe below, or buy in the Spanish section of the supermarket)
3 garlic cloves, peeled and chopped
1 onion, peeled and sliced
1 tablespoon olive oil
2 frying peppers, seeded and chopped
½ cup recaito sauce (*see recipe below, or buy in the Spanish section of the supermarket)
1 cup tomato sauce
2 cups raw long-grain brown rice
5 cups water
15-ounce can pigeon peas (gandules), drained and rinsed
½ cup alcaparrado (green olives, capers, and pimientos, found in the Spanish section of the supermarket)

Cut the chicken breasts into 4-ounce servings. Remove the skin and trim the fat from the chicken legs and thighs. Place the chicken pieces in a bowl and sprinkle the adobo seasoning on the chicken, then stir to coat the chicken. Marinate the chicken in this seasoning in the refrigerator for 1 hour.

Sauté the garlic and onion in the olive oil in a large, heavy pot. Add the chicken and pan-fry on each side for 2 minutes. Remove the chicken from the pot and set aside. Add the frying peppers, recaito, and tomato sauce to the pot. Cook a few minutes.

Rinse the brown rice in a fine mesh strainer to remove some of the starch. Add to the pot along with the water. Cook 30 minutes on medium-low heat, covered. Stir in the pigeon peas and chicken, and cook until the rice absorbs the water. This will take about 20 minutes. Stir in the alcaparrado.

Adobo Powder

> 1 tablespoon garlic powder
> 1 tablespoon onion powder
> 1 tablespoon dried oregano
> ½ tablespoon salt
> 1½ tablespoons black pepper

Mix the ingredients together in a bowl. Store in a plastic bag or small glass jar. Makes 4 tablespoons.

Recaito Sauce

> ½ medium onion, peeled and chopped
> 1 Italian frying pepper, seeded and chopped
> 2 garlic cloves, peeled and chopped
> 3 sweet chili peppers, seeded
> 1 teaspoon chopped cilantro (coriander)

Combine all the ingredients in a blender or food processor. Makes ½ cup. Keep refrigerated.

Makes 8 servings.

Desserts

(Order Based on Prep Time)

1. Mini Strawberry Sundae
2. Really Raspberry Frozen Yogurt
3. Chocolate-Covered Strawberries
4. Baked Fruit Alaska
5. Fruit with Orange Yogurt Sauce
6. Peanut Butter Cookies
7. Mango Custard
8. Basmati Rice Pudding
9. Chocolate Pudding
10. Poached Pears in Red Wine
11. Peach and Blueberry Crisp
12. Flan
13. Peach Frozen Yogurt
14. Creamy Baked Cheesecake with Blueberry Topping

Mini Strawberry Sundae

Prep Time: 5 minutes

This is very satisfying if you have a sweet tooth!

> ½ cup nonfat vanilla frozen yogurt
> 2 strawberries, stems removed and sliced
> 2 tablespoons light chocolate syrup (calorie-reduced syrup)

Place the frozen yogurt in a small bowl. Sprinkle the sliced strawberries around the yogurt.

Squeeze the light syrup on top.

Makes 1 serving.

NUTRITION INFORMATION PER SERVING
Calories: 157
Protein: 5.3 grams
Carbohydrate: 4 grams
Dietary Fiber: 1.3 grams
Fat: 0.5 gram
Saturated Fat: 0.1 gram
Monounsaturated Fat: 0.1 gram
Polyunsaturated Fat: 0.1 gram
Cholesterol: 1.5 milligrams
Sodium: 100 milligrams
Glycemic Index: low

Really Raspberry Frozen Yogurt

Prep Time: 5 minutes

This is soooooo good! Other fruits would work well, too.

> 1 cup frozen raspberries
> 2 cups nonfat vanilla frozen yogurt

Put the raspberries in the food processor and chop for 30 seconds. Spoon in the frozen yogurt, pulse to purée mixture, stopping to scrape the mixture off the processor bowl to better combine the ingredients. Portion out and eat immediately or transfer to a freezer container. Freeze 30 minutes until desired consistency.

Makes 4 servings. Serving size: ½ cup.

NUTRITION INFORMATION PER SERVING
Calories: 123
Protein: 6 grams
Carbohydrate: 25 grams
Dietary Fiber: 1.6 grams
Fat: 0.2 gram
Saturated Fat: 0.1 gram
Monounsaturated Fat: 0 gram
Polyunsaturated Fat: 0 gram
Cholesterol: 1.5 milligrams
Sodium: 65 milligrams
Glycemic Index: low

Chocolate-Covered Strawberries

Prep Time: 10 minutes
Cook Time: 2 minutes

Sometimes the simplest things are the best: delicious rich chocolate covering perfectly ripe strawberries. You don't get a lot, but they are quite satisfying.

20 large strawberries
3 ounces of bittersweet chocolate baking bar

Put the chocolate in a microwave-safe glass bowl and heat on medium-high in the microwave for 2 to 2½ minutes to melt the chocolate. Lay a piece of wax paper or parchment on a baking pan. Stir chocolate with a whisk or fork. Holding the strawberries by the stem, dip them into the chocolate to coat half of the strawberry all around then lay the strawberry on the parchment or waxed paper.

Place in the refrigerator to let the chocolate harden.

Makes 4 servings. Serving size: 5 strawberries.

NUTRITION INFORMATION PER SERVING

Calories: 150
Protein: 2.4 grams
Carbohydrate: 21 grams
Dietary Fiber: 5 grams
Fat: 10 grams
Saturated Fat: 5 grams
Monounsaturated Fat: 0.1 gram
Polyunsaturated Fat: 0.3 gram
Cholesterol: 0 milligram
Sodium: 1 milligram
Glycemic Index: low

Baked Fruit Alaska

Prep Time: 10 minutes
Cook Time: 5 minutes

Fructose is the sugar naturally found in fruit. It is very sweet, so you need to use less fructose than sugar. It is a perfect sweetener for most desserts. You can find it in health food stores and the baking or dietetic section of the supermarket.

1 small ripe cantaloupe
1 cup fresh strawberries, cut up
1 cup blueberries
2 egg whites
pinch of cream of tartar
1 teaspoon fructose or granulated sugar
¼ teaspoon vanilla extract

NUTRITION INFORMATION PER SERVING

Calories: 96
Protein: 3.5 grams
Carbohydrate: 21 grams
Dietary Fiber: 3 grams
Fat: 0.7 gram
Saturated Fat: 0.1 gram
Monounsaturated Fat: 0 gram
Polyunsaturated Fat: 0.3 gram
Cholesterol: 0 milligrams
Sodium: 43 milligrams
Glycemic Index: low

Baked Fruit Alaska (continued)

Preheat broiler. Cut the cantaloupe in half and scoop out seeds. Cut a thin slice from the rounded ends so that cantaloupe halves do not rock when placed on a baking pan. Place the cantaloupe halves on a baking pan. Fill the cantaloupe cavity with the strawberries and blueberries. With a whisk or electric beater, beat the egg whites with the cream of tartar until stiff. Fold in the fructose or sugar and vanilla. Spread the beaten egg whites over the melon halves to completely seal the fruit under a mountain of meringue. Broil for a few minutes until golden brown. Serve at once.

Makes 4 servings. Serving size: ¼ melon.

Fruit with Orange Yogurt Sauce

Prep Time: 15 minutes

Simply arranged and deliciously light.

NUTRITION INFORMATION PER SERVING
Calories: 149
Protein: 4 grams
Carbohydrate: 33 grams
Dietary Fiber: 3.7 grams
Fat: 1.2 grams
Saturated Fat: 0.4 gram
Monounsaturated Fat: 0.2 gram
Polyunsaturated Fat: 3 grams
Cholesterol: 2 milligrams
Sodium: 42 milligrams
Glycemic Index: low

2 kiwis, peeled and sliced
½ ripe medium cantaloupe, cut into bite-size pieces
½ ripe pineapple, peeled, cored, and sliced
8 strawberries, stems removed

Sauce

⅔ cup nonfat plain yogurt
2 tablespoons orange juice concentrate
1 teaspoon vanilla
1 tablespoon honey

Arrange the fruit in a decorative pattern on 4 dessert-size plates. Combine the sauce ingredients in a bowl and stir to make creamy. Drizzle a little sauce on top of the fruit on each plate.

Makes 4 servings.

Peanut Butter Cookies

Prep Time: 10 minutes
Cook Time: 12 minutes

These are great and healthy for you, too. Just don't have more than one. There is no flour in this recipe at all.

1 cup chunky peanut butter
7 tablespoons fructose
1 egg
1 teaspoon baking soda

Preheat oven to 350 degrees. In a mixer, combine all the ingredients. After about a minute, the mixture will get thicker and grainy. Divide cookies into 15 balls; each should be about 1½ inches round. Place on a cookie sheet. Using a fork, press the top of each cookie into a criss-cross pattern to flatten to ½ inch thick. Bake for 10 to 12 minutes until cookies are lightly browned.

Makes 15 cookies. Serving size: 1 cookie.

NUTRITION INFORMATION PER COOKIE

Calories: 129
Protein: 5 grams
Carbohydrate: 9.3 grams
Dietary Fiber: 1.1 grams
Fat: 9 grams
Saturated Fat: 1.8 grams
Monounsaturated Fat: 4.2 grams
Polyunsaturated Fat: 2.5 grams
Cholesterol: 16 milligrams
Sodium: 172 milligrams
Glycemic Index: low

Mango Custard

Prep Time: 10 minutes
Cook Time: 30 minutes

2 cups cubed mango, fresh or frozen-defrosted
2 cups evaporated skim milk
⅓ cup fructose
4 eggs

Preheat oven to 325 degrees. Puree the mango, milk, and fructose in a blender. Transfer to a saucepan and heat over low heat until the mixture comes to a low simmer. Remove from heat and let cool for a few minutes. Mix the eggs in a bowl, then pour them into the cooled mango mixture. Pour this mixture into 8 porcelain ramekins.

NUTRITION INFORMATION PER SERVING

Calories: 152
Protein: 9 grams
Carbohydrate: 23 grams
Dietary Fiber: 0.7 gram
Fat: 3 grams
Saturated Fat: 1 gram
Monounsaturated Fat: 1.2 grams
Polyunsaturated Fat: 0.4 gram
Cholesterol: 126 milligrams
Sodium: 111 milligrams
Glycemic Index: low

Mango Custard (continued)

Put the ramekins in a baking pan large enough to hold them; the pan should have 2-inch sides. Pour enough water around the ramekins into the pan so that the water comes halfway up the outside of each ramekin. Bake for 25 minutes or until center is firm to touch.

Makes 8 servings.

Basmati Rice Pudding

Prep Time: 5 minutes
Cook Time: 35 minutes

1½ cups water
1 cup white basmati rice
2 cups skim milk
1 teaspoon vanilla extract
1 cinnamon stick
5 tablespoons fructose
2 egg yolks, stirred
Cinnamon to sprinkle on top

NUTRITION INFORMATION PER SERVING:

Calories: 158
Protein: 5 grams
Carbohydrate: 31 grams
Dietary Fiber: 0.2 gram
Fat: 1.6 grams
Saturated Fat: 0.5 gram
Monounsaturated Fat: 0.6 gram
Polyunsaturated Fat: 0.3 gram
Cholesterol: 54 milligrams
Sodium: 37 milligrams
Glycemic Index: low

Bring the water to a boil in a saucepan. Add the rice, reduce heat to low, and cook for 10 minutes. Add the milk, vanilla extract, cinnamon stick, and fructose and cook, covered, on low for 15 more minutes, stirring occasionally. Make sure the heat is on low so that you don't scorch the pudding. Remove lid, stir in the yolks, and continue stirring as the mixture thickens. Pour into a serving bowl or 8 small bowls to cool. Cover with plastic wrap. Sprinkle a little cinnamon on top before serving.

Makes 8 servings. Serving size: ½ cup.

Chocolate Pudding

Prep and Cook Time: 15 minutes
Refrigeration Time: 30 minutes

2 cups skim milk
⅓ cup granulated sugar
5 tablespoons cocoa powder
3 tablespoons cornstarch

NUTRITION
INFORMATION PER
SERVING
Calories: 148
Protein: 6 grams
Carbohydrate: 32 grams
Dietary Fiber: 2.3 grams
Fat: 1 gram
Saturated Fat: 0.5 gram
Monounsaturated Fat: 0
    gram
Polyunsaturated Fat: 0
    gram
Cholesterol: 2 milligrams
Sodium: 67 milligrams
Glycemic Index: low

In a heavy pot, combine 1½ cups of the milk, the sugar and cocoa. Using a whisk, stir until lump-free over low heat. In a separate cup, mix the remaining ½ cup of skim milk with the cornstarch until lump-free. Stir the cornstarch mixture into the pot and cook, bring to a boil and cook an additional 3–5 minutes. Spoon pudding into individual serving bowls. Refrigerate until cool, about 30 minutes.

Makes 4 servings.

Poached Pears in Red Wine

Prep Time: 10 minutes
Cook Time: 40 minutes

Always a refreshing sweet!

8 small ripe pears
1 cup apple juice concentrate
½ cup burgundy-type wine
1 teaspoon vanilla extract
1 cup water

NUTRITION
INFORMATION PER
SERVING
Calories: 141
Protein: 0.7 gram
Carbohydrate: 33 grams
Dietary Fiber: 3.5 grams
Fat: 0.6 gram
Saturated Fat: 0 gram
Monounsaturated Fat:
    0.1 gram
Polyunsaturated Fat: 0.2
    gram
Cholesterol: 0 milligram
Sodium: 8 milligrams
Glycemic Index: low

Peel and core the pears. Combine the apple juice, wine, vanilla, and water in a pot. Bring to a simmer and add the pears. Cook on medium-low for 20 to 30 minutes, turning halfway if the pears are not completely covered with liquid. (Cover with a lid for faster cooking.) Remove the pears from the pot and set aside. Cook the remaining liquid at a low simmer for 10 more minutes to make a syrup. Serve pears with a little syrup drizzled on top.

Makes 8 servings. Serving size: 1 pear.

Peach and Blueberry Crisp

Prep Time: 15 minutes
Cook Time: 35 minutes

3 peaches, halved, pitted, peeled, and sliced, about
   3 cups
1 cup fresh blueberries
2 tablespoons fructose
1 teaspoon freshly grated lemon peel
½ teaspoon ground cinnamon
¼ teaspoon ground nutmeg (optional)
1 tablespoon unbleached wheat flour or cornstarch

Topping

½ cup old-fashioned rolled oats
1 tablespoon whole-wheat or white unbleached flour
3 tablespoons fructose
½ teaspoon ground cinnamon
2 tablespoons cold butter

NUTRITION INFORMATION PER SERVING

Calories: 160
Protein: 33 grams
Carbohydrate: 31 grams
Dietary Fiber: 4 grams
Fat: 4 grams
Saturated Fat: 2.2 grams
Monounsaturated Fat: 0.1 gram
Polyunsaturated Fat: 0.1 gram
Cholesterol: 8 milligrams
Sodium: 3 milligrams
Glycemic Index: low

Preheat oven to 350 degrees. In a bowl, mix the peaches, blueberries, fructose, lemon peel, cinnamon, nutmeg, and flour. Transfer the peach and blueberry mixture into an 8-by-8-inch baking pan.

In a separate bowl, mix the oats, whole-wheat or white flour, fructose, and cinnamon. Cut the butter or margarine into small pieces, then mix it quickly into the oat mixture with your hands. The mixture will be coarse and crumbly. Pour the oat mixture on top of the peaches. Bake for 35 minutes.

Makes 6 servings.

Flan

Prep Time: 20 minutes
Cook Time: 50 minutes

Flan is a baked custard. It is easy to make, creamy, and delicious.

¼ cup granulated sugar
4 whole eggs
2½ cups evaporated skim milk
⅓ cup fructose powder
1 teaspoon vanilla extract

Preheat oven to 325 degrees. In a saucepan, heat the sugar until it browns and caramelizes. Pour this into the center of the bottom of an 8-inch round cake pan or glass dish. It will harden immediately. Set aside.

Beat the eggs with a whisk in a bowl. Stir in the milk, fructose, and vanilla. Mix until well combined. Pour over the caramelized sugar in the pan.

Place this pan in a larger pan with sides, and pour water around the larger pan so that the water comes about halfway up the outside of the flan pan. Bake for 50 minutes. Remove from heat. Let cool slightly. Using a small knife, cut gently between the flan and the pan to release. Put a plate on top of the pan and flip both to release the flan onto the plate. Cut into 8 pieces.

Makes 8 servings.

NUTRITION INFORMATION PER SERVING
Calories: 157
Protein: 10 grams
Carbohydrate: 22 grams
Dietary Fiber: 0 gram
Fat: 3 grams
Saturated Fat: 1 gram
Monounsaturated Fat: 1.2 grams
Polyunsaturated Fat: 0.4 gram
Cholesterol: 127 milligrams
Sodium: 130 milligrams
Glycemic Index: low

Peach Frozen Yogurt

Prep Time: 10 minutes
Freezer Time: 2 hours

10 ounces frozen peaches
1 cup nonfat vanilla yogurt
2 tablespoons fructose

Place the peaches, yogurt, and fructose in the food processor and puree until well combined. If you have an ice-cream maker, transfer the peach-yogurt mixture to the ice-cream maker and follow the manufacturer's instructions. If you don't have one, transfer the puree to a plastic container and freeze for about 2 hours, stirring every half hour.

Makes 4 servings.

NUTRITION INFORMATION PER SERVING

Calories: 94
Protein: 3 grams
Carbohydrate: 21 grams
Dietary Fiber: 1 gram
Fat: 0 gram
Saturated Fat: 0 gram
Monounsaturated Fat: 0 gram
Polyunsaturated Fat: 0 gram
Cholesterol: 1 milligram
Sodium: 33 milligrams
Glycemic Index: low

Creamy Baked Cheesecake with Blueberry Topping

Prep Time: 15 minutes
Cook Time: 40 minutes
Refrigeration Time: 2 hours

This cake is so good and healthy that you could have a leftover piece for breakfast!

2 cups 1%-fat cottage cheese
3 ounces low-fat cream cheese
2 eggs
2 teaspoons grated lemon rind
6 tablespoons fructose
1 teaspoon vanilla extract

Topping

2 cups fresh or frozen blueberries
1 tablespoon cornstarch
1½ tablespoons fructose

NUTRITION INFORMATION PER SERVING

Calories: 127
Protein: 10 grams
Carbohydrate: 13 grams
Dietary Fiber: 1 gram
Fat: 4 grams
Saturated Fat: 2 grams
Monounsaturated Fat: 1.3 grams
Polyunsaturated Fat: 0.3 gram
Cholesterol: 70 milligrams
Sodium: 282 milligrams
Glycemic Index: low

Preheat oven to 325 degrees.

Purée the cottage cheese, cream cheese, and eggs in a food processor or blender until smooth. Add the lemon rind, fructose, and vanilla and purée to combine. Pour mixture into a 7- or 8-inch round springform pan. Place the springform pan in a round pan that is slightly larger and pour water around the outside of the springform pan into the larger pan. Place in the oven and bake for 40 minutes. The center should be firm to the touch.

Remove the pans from the oven and let sit 30 minutes to cool.

Combine the blueberries, cornstarch, and fructose in a bowl suitable for the microwave.

Microwave on high for 3 minutes. Stir, then microwave 2 more minutes. Remove from oven and let cool for 5 minutes.

Cut around the outside of the pan before releasing. Place the cheesecake in the springform pan onto a dinner plate. After the cooked berry mixture has cooled, spoon it onto the top of the cake. Refrigerate until serving. Cut into 8 pieces.

Makes 8 servings.

Appendix
Glycemic Index Chart

	GI
Pastries/Cake/Dairy	
Angel Food Cake	Medium
Banana Cake	Medium
Carrot Cake	Medium
Cupcake	High
Doughnut	High
Ice Cream	Medium
Milk	Low
Pie Crust	Medium
Pound Cake	Medium
Pudding (no starch)	Low
Pudding, Tapioca	High
Scones	High
Sponge Cake	Low
Yogurt (plain)	Low
Breads/Crackers/Cookies	
Bagel	High
Blueberry Muffin	Medium
Bran Muffin	Medium
Corn Muffin	High
Crackers	High
Croissant	Medium
English Muffin	High
French Bread	High
Flour Cookies	High
Graham Crackers	High
Hamburger Bun	Medium

	GI
Hot Dog Bun	Medium
Kaiser Roll	High
Melba Toast	High
Multigrain Bread	Low
Oatmeal Cookies	Low
Pancakes/Waffles	High
Pita Bread	Medium
Pumpernickel	Low
Rice Cakes	High
Rye Bread	Low
Sourdough Bread	Low
Taco Shells	High
Vanilla Wafers	High
White Bread	High
Whole-Wheat Bread	Medium
Whole-Wheat Stone Ground	Low
Potatoes/Rice/Barley/Pasta	
Barley	Low
Potato, Baked	High
Potato, Mashed	High
Potato, French Fry	High
Potato, New	Medium
Potato, Sweet	Low
Potato, Yam	Low
Rice, Brown	Low
Rice, Converted	Low
Rice, Short Grain	High

	GI		GI
Rice, Instant	High	Kidney Beans	Low
Rice, Wild	Medium	Lentils	Low
Pasta, Fettuccine	Low	Lettuce	Low
Pasta, Linguini	Low	Lima Beans	Low
Pasta, Macaroni	Low	Mushrooms	Low
Pasta, Mac and Cheese	Medium	Navy Beans	Low
Pasta, Ravioli	Low	Onions	Low
Pasta, Spaghetti	Low	Parsnips	High
		Peas	Low
Fruit		Peppers	Low
		Red Beans	Low
Apple	Low	Spinach	Low
Apple Juice	Low	String Beans	Low
Apricot	Medium	Tomato	Low
Banana	Medium		
Cantaloupe	Medium	*Cereal*	
Cherries	Low		
Cranberry Juice	Medium	All-Bran	Low
Figs, Dried	Medium	Bran Chex	Medium
Fruit Cocktail	Medium	Bran Flakes	High
Grapefruit	Low	Cheerios	High
Grapefruit Juice	Low	Corn Chex	High
Grapes	Low	Cornflakes	High
Kiwi	Medium	Corn Pops	High
Mango	Low	Cream of Wheat	High
Orange	Low	Fruit Loops	Medium
Orange Juice	Medium	Frosted Flakes	Medium
Peach	Low	Life	Medium
Pears	Low	Mini Wheats	Medium
Pineapple	Medium	Muesli	Low
Pineapple Juice	Low	Oat Bran	Low
Plum	Low	Oatmeal, Instant	Medium
Prune	Low	Oatmeal, Regular	Low
Raisins	Medium	Puffed Rice	High
Strawberry	Low	Puffed Wheat	Medium
Watermelon	High	Raisin Bran	Medium
		Rice Krispies	High
Vegetables/Beans		Shredded Wheat	High
		Special K	Medium
Baked Beans	Low	Total	High
Beets	Medium		
Black-eyed Peas	Low	*Snacks*	
Cabbage	Low		
Carrots	Low	Coke	High
Cauliflower	Low	Corn Chips	High
Chickpeas	Low	Fructose	Low

	GI		GI
Gatorade	High	Pretzels	High
Honey	Medium	Protein Bars	Low
Mars Bar	Medium	Protein Shakes	Low
M&Ms, Peanut	Low	Skittles	High
Nuts	Low	Snickers Bar	High
Popcorn	Medium	Sugar, Table (sucrose)	Medium
Potato Chips	High		

Index

You are invited

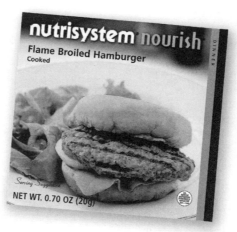

nutrisystem nourish
Flame Broiled Hamburger
Cooked

NET WT. 0.70 OZ (20g)

We invite you to experience

how truly wonderful the NutriSystem

Nourish Prepared Foods Meal Plan is and

to enjoy free shipping with your first order.